PANDORA PRESS

YOUR BOI
YOUR BAI
YOUR LIFL

Angela Phillips is a journalist, photographer, author, feminist and mother. She was the co-editor of the very successful UK edition of *Our Bodies, Ourselves* and writes widely for the national newspapers and women's magazines. *Your Body, Your Baby, Your Life* is her first book, written out of interest and concern arising from her own experience of childbirth, the women's movement and trade union involvement. Angela Phillips took the photograph on the front cover of this book.

Angela Phillips was assisted in writing *Your Body, Your Baby, Your Life* by Nicky Lean and Barbara Jacobs.

Nicky Lean has worked for many years as a childbirth teacher for the National Childbirth Trust and has recently completed her midwifery training. She is a member of the Association of Radical Midwives and has three children.

Barbara Jacobs qualified in medicine in 1970; she worked in hospital medicine for five years before setting up in general practice. She has always had a special concern for women's health, obstetrics and women patients' rights.

YOUR BODY, YOUR BABY, YOUR LIFE takes you all the way from six months before conception, through pregnancy and birth and stays with you until you are safely into the new world of parenthood.

YOUR BODY, YOUR BABY, YOUR LIFE

Angela Phillips
with Nicky Lean and Barbara Jacobs

Illustrated by Ros Asquith

PANDORA PRESS
London, Melbourne and Henley

First published in 1983
by Pandora Press
(Routledge & Kegan Paul, plc)
39 Store Street, London WC1E 7DD, England
464 St Kilda Road, Melbourne,
Victoria 3004, Australia and
Broadway House, Newtown Road,
Henley-on-Thames, Oxon RG9 1EN, England
Set in Century by Input Typesetting Ltd, London
and printed in Great Britain by Unwin Brothers Ltd,
Old Woking, Surrey

British Library Cataloguing in Publication Data

Phillips, Angela

Your body, your baby, your life.
1. Pregnancy   2. Childbirth
I. Title   II. Lean, Nicky III. Jacobs, Barbara
618.2'00240431   RG525

ISBN 0–86358–006–8

CONTENTS

INTRODUCTION

This is the book I wanted to read when I was pregnant. There was plenty to read about birth but for the nine months before and after, I felt very much on my own. Books did exist but they were written for a strange breed of women who did nothing during pregnancy except make themselves pretty for their husbands, and nothing afterwards except look after their babies. These books were not about me.

The practical information about pregnancy was either incomplete or hedged about with unacceptable notions about the dangers of listening to other women and the importance of accepting what your doctor tells you. My experience, in the women's health movement, had long ago warned me that doctors are not always right and that they do not always even listen. I needed the information which would make it possible to participate intelligently in my own antenatal care.

After the birth I was forced to resort to books which doled out dollops of guilt with the advice on nappies and feeding. Nothing I could find was encouraging about my particular concerns as a mother who needed to earn a living. These books didn't begin to prepare me for the changes which parenthood would bring.

I cannot be the only woman to feel this lack. For most women today, pregnancy and childbirth is *the* initiation into adulthood. As young women we lead independent, active lives, with or without partners. Parenthood changes that utterly. However close we may have come to achieving equality in our working and personal lives before having children, afterwards we have been brought up very sharply against the fact that, in our society, equality is for childless women.

In the ten years since the British parliament decreed that pregnant women should have a right to job security and maternity leave, women's needs and aspirations have been changing. Those of us who believe that having a baby should not mean drawing a curtain on our former lives and outside interests are no longer isolated individuals. So far we have not had the time to gather, and share experience about the best way to manage our lives. Everyone is going through the same hoops making the same mistakes.

This book brings some of that information together. It combines explanations about what is happening to our bodies with comments from women who have themselves lived through these changes. It is not about shoulds, and oughts, but a sharing of experience as varied as any kitchen table discussion amongst women who have borne children. Some women talk with a glow of pride about giving birth, others (me included) feel we could do better next time.

The biggest contributions come from Nicky Lean and Barbara Jacobs both as mothers and health workers who have held many women's hands during pregnancy and labour. But every other woman I know who has been pregnant will find a little piece of herself in here. I owe thanks to them all but special thanks must go to the Doddington Women's Group, who kept my head above water, Riva Klein, Tessa Turner, Sue Barlow, Penny Valentine, Sara Harrison, Marianne Scruggs, Wendy Farrant, Penny Vincenzi, Katie Simmons, Miriam Beeks, and to Nicky's NCT classes.

Chapter 1

BEFORE THE BEGINNING

Few of us plan our pregnancies so carefully that we would read a book about it beforehand. And yet we are beginning to discover that the first days in the life of a developing human being may be the most important in terms of its future health. That means that your health, and your partner's, is as important at the moment of conception as at the moment of birth.

Of course even tip-top health won't make any of us immune to the heartbreak of a handicapped baby, but gradually information is being collected which can help us to safeguard our babies. Some of the most important factors are quite beyond our control. Living in a polluted environment, handling dangerous chemicals at work and having no access to shops which stock a good range of fresh foods put anyone at a disadvantage in looking after their own health. However, even if you cannot reduce pollution or equalise wages overnight, you can take steps to protect yourself, particularly before and during pregnancy.

Eating right

'The most important period for nutritional care appears to be in the few weeks before and immediately after conception. This is not usually the time when diet is considered important,'

writes pathologist Isobel Jennings, while Dr William Rogers of Texas University goes even further:

'If all prospective human mothers could be fed as expertly as prospective animal mothers in the laboratory, most sterility, spontaneous abortions and premature births would disappear; the birth of deformed and mentally retarded babies would be largely a thing of the past.'

Food isn't just fuel, it provides the basic building bricks of life.
You can build a house with almost anything, but if you use good
materials it will last longer, work better and need fewer repairs.
So it is with people. Though Dr Rogers may be slightly overstat-
ing his case (after all infections of the fallopian tubes are probably an equally important cause of sterility), some studies both
here and abroad have shown that the rate of birth abnormalities
and certain complications in pregnancy drop when dietary supplements are given to women at risk before and during
pregnancy.

A healthy diet must include not only the basics: carbo-
hydrate, protein and fats, but also the invisible foods: vitamins,
trace elements and minerals. Taking a few vitamin pills along
with a bad diet may not be enough to make the difference. Good
eating lies in balance. Foods work together and must be eaten
together if they are to do their work properly. Experiments have
shown that, when all the different vitamins in the 'B' complex
were given to rats, 80 per cent of them were resistant to disease
whereas only 20 per cent of those supplied with an incomplete
set of B vitamins survived.

Minerals are also part of the complex chain your body needs
if it is to work efficiently. You need iron in your blood to guard
against anaemia; one place you will find iron is in eggs, but your
body won't use it properly without vitamin C which you find in
most fruits and many vegetables. Similarly, you need vitamin B
to make use of the energy in sugar if your brain is to function
well. Vitamin B6 (just one of the B vitamins) in turn needs a
touch of the trace element zinc. Some vitamins can be taken in
quite large quantities because the extra will simply be washed
away in your urine. On the other hand, fat soluble vitamins such
as vitamins A and D can be stored, and overdosing may actually
be dangerous. If you come from Asia you may need extra vitamin
D to make up for our lack of sunshine. This vitamin comes in
dairy products, eggs and fish. So if you eat none of those, you
may need a supplement of vitamin D. Ask your doctor.

If all this sounds horribly complicated don't worry, the answer doesn't lie in memorising a diet sheet. It lies in eating food
in a state which is as close as possible to the way it grew, so that
it contains most of its own vitamins and minerals. The more
refined a food becomes, i.e. the more factory processes which lie
between it and you, the more will be lost.

Do eat something raw every day. Most fruits and vegetables (excluding potatoes) may be eaten raw, alone or mixed in salads. You can try adding a little of the raw vegetable, chopped fine, to cooked vegetables just before serving.

Eat wholemeal bread, crispbreads and cereals. In every case make sure it really is *whole* and not just brown. Muesli, Weetabix, Shreddies, Shredded Wheat and porridge are all made from whole grains. Highly refined foods like cornflakes and white bread lack not only the necessary minerals and trace elements but also the roughage which keeps your digestive system in working order.

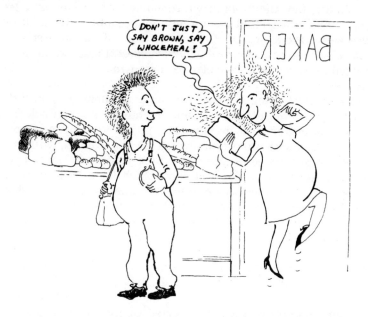

Avoid eating foods which are highly processed: sugar or anything made mainly from sugar (where ingredients are listed on the package, the largest ingredient always comes first); white flour, or anything made mainly with white flour (white bread, cakes, biscuits, etc.); tinned fruits and vegetables which are preserved in sugar and stripped of much of their food value through processing; potatoes which have turned green in the frost (they contain poisonous nitrates); or any mouldy foods. Avoid as far as possible any foods which say on the packaging that they contain preservatives (including tinned and preserved meats).

These are all unbalanced foods which either do not contain

the vitamins and minerals necessary for proper use, or do contain chemicals which could be damaging to health. Sugar is particularly bad. It is such a concentrated food (the average daily intake in this country is about equivalent to eating 2½ lbs of sugar beet daily), that it requires large quantities of vitamins and minerals if it is to be broken down. It therefore uses up all of these vitamins it can find in the body and leaves you deficient. We don't really need to eat sugar at all. Our bodies will manufacture it from fruit and vegetables, but unfortunately many of us are addicted to it and find it very hard to give up. So it's worth remembering that in Britain and Ireland we consume more sugar and less fresh fruit and vegetables than any other country in the developed world. We also have the highest rate of babies born with spina bifida. If, as some researchers suspect, these two facts are connected, we have a very strong reason indeed to change our eating habits.

Food tips   Steam vegetables or cook them in very little water to preserve the water-soluble vitamins B and C. Cook fruit in iron, enamel or glass, because aluminium saucepans can contaminate food with aluminium which is to be avoided, while iron saucepans contribute usable iron which you need. Try to eat a fair amount of vegetables and fruit which have been grown in this country. Fresh foods contain more vitamins than ones which have been stored. If you eat imported foods you can be certain that they have been stored and they have probably been ripened artificially too.

Hazards at work

Both men and women can be affected by industrial substances which cause infertility, spontaneous abortions, stillbirth or malformed babies.

In the lead and radiation industries, these hazards are recognized and exposure levels have been set, often allowing men greater exposure than women, with special low levels for pregnant women. In fact, setting different levels of exposure is pointless. Sperm which are being constantly manufactured in the testes (balls) are in need of equal protection. A poisonous substance could cause sterility or impotence or damage the sperm enough to cause miscarriage, stillbirth or possibly abnormalities. Similarly, providing special protection for pregnant women is of little use if they are exposed to higher levels in the early days before realising that they are pregnant, when the foetus is at its most vulnerable.

Unfortunately insufficient research has been carried out into the effects of industrial pollutants on human reproduction. In some cases, animal experiments have been done, but the information has not always been applied to setting safety levels for people. One pesticide called Dibromchloropropane (DBPC) was known to have a bad effect on male animal reproduction. It wasn't until men working in the plant started comparing notes that they realised it also caused sterility in humans. The pesticide is no longer manufactured in the West, but its record didn't stop industrialists exporting the chemical plant to a Third World country where regulations are less stringent.

Your rights   Under the terms of the Congenital Disabilities (Civil Liabilities) Act your employer could be sued if your child was born with a malformation which could be traced to your place of work. This law applies to malformations carried through either the mother or the father. Nevertheless you won't want to wait until the damage is done. Get your trade union health and safety representative to look into the substances you are working with. They should then argue with your employer for either the removal of known hazards or better safety precautions. Their best weapon in this argument is to point out the potential expense of defending cases under the Congenital Disabilities Act as well as the possibility of heavy compensation.

Once you are pregnant, you have a right to be moved to a safer job under the terms of the Employment Protection Act which prevents your employer from sacking you because of your pregnancy. However, as your growing baby is at its most vulnerable in the first few days of its life, before you are certain you actually are pregnant, changing your job in advance is a safer bet if you work with a known hazardous substance.

Some known hazardous substances are aniline, benzene, toluene, carbon monoxide, polychlorinated byphenyls, Hexachlorabenzene, inorganic lead, organic mercury, radioactive substances and X-rays (from a US Department of Labour list compiled in 1942).

Other known or strongly suspected hazards to fertility and reproduction are anaesthetic gases (many hospitals now use special extractor fans to cut down on waste products), vinyl chloride (PVC) (exposure levels to this substance have been dropped to a safer level after ICI was forced to pay out substantial damages to workers), oestrogens, pesticides containing organochlorines and dioxin (workers using pesticides are as vulnerable as those who manufacture them if adequate safety precautions are not observed), carbon disulphide (used in the manufacture of viscose rayons), phthalate plasticisers, boric acid and formaldeyhide.

This might seem like a long list, but it's a mere drop in the ocean of the estimated 100,000 substances in industrial use. Threshold limit values (TLVs) indicating the safe level of exposure have been set for only 500 of them, and even these do not necessarily take reproductive risks into account. The rest will remain unknown quantities until workers, comparing notes, discover their dangers.

Breaking the habits

Smoking Smokers run a greater risk of miscarrying and their babies may be lighter than normal at birth. Low birth weight babies are more vulnerable to a range of possible difficulties starting life and are more likely to need 'special care'. Smoking may also affect male fertility. Smoke breathed in by a pregnant woman from other smokers will also reach the baby. Apart from the direct effects of smoking, cigarettes also rob the mother's body of vital vitamins and minerals which are necessary to the healthy development of the baby, causing a kind of malnutrition.

Kicking this habit can be hard. Start well in advance. Pregnancy can be difficult enough without the added complication of withdrawal symptoms from giving up smoking. Some Area Health Authorities provide special anti-smoking clinics or support groups. Ask your doctor for help, or contact ASH (see page 203).

Alcohol is another common poison which can damage a developing baby. Researchers have grouped together its effects under the name foetal alcohol syndrome. The main danger is mental handicap. There is no clearly safe drinking level. Some say you should give it up altogether, others that only heavy bouts of drinking will have an effect. Like smoking, alcohol robs the body of vital nutrients which should be better used. In particular heavy drinkers tend to lack vitamins B and C.

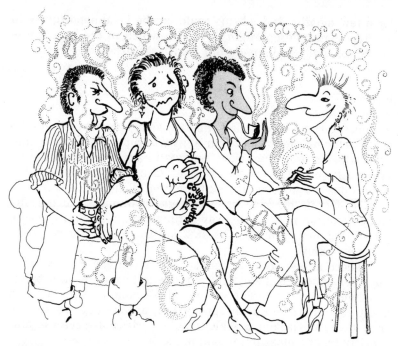

Since alcohol can affect the baby at the very earliest stage of development, it would be prudent to cut down as much as possible in advance of pregnancy. Once you are pregnant, your body may become your biggest ally. Many pregnant women find that they cannot stand the taste of alcohol.

If you are frightened at the thought of life without a drink, you may need help giving it up. Contact DAWN (see page 203) or Alcoholics Anonymous. Wanting a baby may be the spur you need to come to terms with this habit.

The Pill cannot really be classified as a habit, but it is a good idea to stop taking it a few months before you start trying to get pregnant. Women on the Pill are very often deficient in vitamin B6 (pyridoxine) (found in wholemeal bread and yeast), an important nutrient for a healthy pregnancy. It isn't a bad idea also to give your body time to get rid of the synthetic hormones in the Pill. Doses of similar hormones, prescribed in large quantities during pregnancy in the past, have since been associated with cancer in children, so it is wise to be cautious.

Once you've decided to plan ahead for a child, you will probably be happy to use a slightly less effective birth control method for a few months. Indeed this could be the ideal opportunity to practise using a diaphragm or sheath which in the long run is much less likely to damage your health than the Pill.

Exercise

Exercising won't have much effect on your baby's health, but it could make a difference to your ability to cope in pregnancy and after. During pregnancy your body will have to get used to carrying a lot of extra weight around. Once the baby is born the weight doesn't go away. It gets bigger daily and still wants to be carried. Gentle exercise such as yoga, swimming and dancing can be kept up most of the way through pregnancy. It's wise to get started now so that by the time you are pregnant it will have become a habit.

There is one special exercise which you can do any time, anywhere, starting today. Its purpose is to tone up the pelvic floor muscles around your vagina. These muscles come under a great deal of strain during labour and, unless they are kept in trim, they can slacken. Slack vaginal muscles may decrease your sensitivity, and pleasure, in making love.

To find them, try stopping and starting the flow when you next have a pee, by squeezing and relaxing. Those are the muscles. Exercise them by slowly contracting and relaxing them ten times every time you remember to do it.

Medical checks

Rubella, or German measles as it is more commonly known, is a very mild disease which can sometimes pass unnoticed and yet it can do enormous damage to a developing baby in those first twelve weeks of pregnancy. Your doctor can give you a blood test to discover whether you are immune to the disease. If you are not, you may be vaccinated against it. Take great care not to get pregnant for three months so that the vaccine itself won't damage the baby.

Drugs, both on prescription and off, have been implicated in causing birth defects. Now is the time to talk to your doctor about the possibility of reducing your dosage, or coming off long-term drug treatments altogether. Epileptics would do well to seek referral to a neurologist to discuss the best way of handling a pregnancy and anyone with heart or kidney disease should also discuss treatment with a doctor in advance of pregnancy.

Tests for anaemia, VD and diabetes are always done at ante-natal clinics once you are pregnant. It would of course be better to deal with any problems like this before you actually get pregnant. Your doctor will probably be quite happy to do the necessary blood and urine tests if you explain why you want them. If there is any chance that either of you could be carrying even a mild form of sexually transmitted disease, do get yourself checked, and treated. These infections can still be treated during pregnancy but it's worth avoiding the necessity for taking large doses of antibiotics which could be absorbed by your developing baby.

Genetic counselling is available at every major teaching hospital. If you are concerned about a handicap which appears to be passed on through your families, you can ask your doctor to refer you for genetic counselling. The counsellor will help you discover whether the problem is, in fact, inherited, what your chances are of passing it on, and whether tests are available to diagnose it during pregnancy.

Planning ahead at work

'I was really looking forward to leaving work and staying home full time with my baby, but now I'm actually doing it I'm bored and miserable and would give anything to get my job back.'

It is hard to imagine in advance whether or not you'll want to return to work once your baby is born. Some women make elaborate plans for keeping their jobs open and then find themselves so wrapped up in their new babies that they resign before their maternity leave ends. But around 40 per cent of those women in paid work during their pregnancies are actually back or looking for employment by the time their babies are eight months old. The percentage grows bigger the older their children grow. So it's worth finding out in advance just what your rights actually are. The law is explained more fully in chapter 3.

Your trade union may well have negotiated an improved maternity leave agreement with your employer. Find out what, if anything, has been done. Some unions have won a shorter qualifying period (say one year) or none at all, for the right to job reinstatement. Others have gone much further and obtained longer periods of paid leave, the right to return to work on a part-time basis for the first few weeks, or a much longer-term right to job reinstatement.

If you are not satisfied with your current maternity agreement now is the time to argue for improvements. Talk to your trade union representative at work. Constructive interest from members is usually welcomed. You may like to arm yourself with more information on current agreements, so read *Maternity Rights for Working Women* or *Bargaining Report 8* (see page 201).

If there is no union at your work place, you could speak to your personnel manager, or equivalent, but take care, the Employment Protection Act prevents your employer sacking you if you are pregnant, but it gives you no protection from dismissal for considering pregnancy.

Planning ahead at home

Britain is suffering from a housing crisis. Current government policies of selling off council houses are reducing housing stocks still further and making it worse. None the less, a pregnant woman, or a woman with a child, is entitled to some sort of roof under the terms of the Housing (Homeless Persons) Act 1977. This is by no means an easy route to a home. In many areas you will be expected to live in cramped bed and breakfast accommodation or hostels for many months before being allocated a flat and even then you will have virtually no right to choose the kind of home you might wish for yourself.

If you are considering moving to a larger place, it is worthwhile trying to do it before you get pregnant. Of course few of us are actually that far-sighted, but anyone who has actually tried to sort out their housing problems towards the end of pregnancy, or with a small baby, will testify to the difficulty.

'We had only one room which was warm, safe and clean, even a trip to the bathroom was a bit hazardous, what with floor boards pulled up and tools all over the place. He was miserable and clung to me. I was frantic and isolated. I fervently wished we had moved before I got pregnant.'

PROBLEMS GETTING PREGNANT

About one in every eight couples have not conceived after a year of trying. Half of them will achieve pregnancy without any help and a further 15–20 per cent can be helped medically.

Causes of infertility vary but it's probable that in about 30 per cent of cases, the problems will be joint ones and of the rest, half can be traced to the man and half to the woman.

Joint problems

Sexual difficulties For a woman to get pregnant, the sperm has to be delivered near to the neck of her womb at the right time of the month. If the man is unable to achieve this or the couple don't enjoy sex enough to make love sufficiently frequently, sperm and egg may never meet. If the couple don't feel inclined to get to the root of the sexual difficulties, the sperm can be collected in a test tube and inserted, at the right time, and to the right place, artificially. Otherwise a menstrual chart, available from family planning clinics, may help you find your fertile time.

An infection called T Mycoplasma may be preventing pregnancy. It can be treated with antibiotics.

An allergic reaction to sperm may produce antibodies which destroy them.

Women's problems

Temporary infertility may be caused by the contraceptive pill or injection. There is no evidence that the Pill causes permanent sterility though it isn't yet possible to be quite certain of the long-term effect of contraceptive injections.

Overwork, exhaustion, stress and a bad diet can all affect your ability to conceive and you can treat them all yourself. Check also that you are not working with any of the chemicals listed on page 5.

Psychological problems may be to blame. Some people just don't conceive until they've given up hope. Probably the best treatment for this is to find something else to absorb your attention. It is also the most difficult thing to do.

Internal obstructions can be caused by infections which, if not treated swiftly enough, may cause scabs to form on the tubes, so that they stick together and block the passage of the egg back into the womb. These blockages may be removed surgically, or, if the tubes are too badly damaged, they may sometimes be replaced or mended with microsurgery, but such techniques are not always successful.

Abnormal growths of the womb lining, such as fibroids, inside the womb, or endometriosis outside, can also hinder the process of fertilisation and implantation. In both cases surgery may be necessary to remove the scar tissue.

Hormones are touchy things and, if they have been upset, a drug may be prescribed to jolt them back to work. These drugs have caused multiple births, but doses are rather better controlled these days.

Men's problems

Temporary infertility may be caused by heat: give up hot baths, invest in looser underwear and pack away your tight jeans. A very hot working environment, an inadequate diet and smoking can also inhibit sperm production.

Tube damage may have been caused by illness such as TB, mumps (in an adult) or other infections. A physical abnormality may also block the tubes. Microsurgery may be able to mend the damage but it isn't always successful.

Dangerous substances at work could be to blame. They can affect the number and mobility (movement) of sperm.

Hormones may also be a factor, in which case drug treatment may be necessary.

Getting help

Your doctor can refer you to a sub-fertility clinic. You may need to wait for some time for an appointment and the testing can be drawn out over many months. The process may have a shattering effect on your relationship. You may find yourself organising your sex life around dates on a calendar, rather than according to whim or desire. When sex becomes a chore, or just a means to an end, it is hard to find ways to comfort each other. This is a

time when you both need comfort, and even though finding someone to talk to will probably help, it may not be easy to find a
sympathetic listener.

The books mentioned on page 201 may give you some useful
advice on what you can expect at the clinics.

Artificial insemination by donor

If your partner is infertile, or there is no man in your life with
whom you would want to embark on pregnancy, then AID may
be a route to motherhood.

If you are considering AID as a couple it is very important
to get proper counselling and ensure that the feelings of both of
you about it are well aired. If you are single, or in a lesbian
relationship, you will probably have done a great deal of hard
thinking to get this far.

An infertility clinic will refer you for AID or, if you are not
attending a clinic, you could ask your GP for a referral to one.
Single or lesbian women will do better contacting the British
Pregnancy Advisory Service (see page 203) for counselling and
'treatment' or finding a donor and doing it yourselves.

Self-insemination has been pioneered by lesbian women. In
the past, lesbians wanting to have babies have usually been
forced into unwanted, and often unhappy, relationships with men
to achieve their aim. As many are now finding, to their cost, any
attempt to separate from the father at a later stage can result in
loss, not only of custody but, in some cases even of visiting rights.
AID avoids these problems. A pamphlet called 'Self Insemination'
explains what to do (see page 201).

Chapter 2

OVER THE MOON OR UNDER THE WEATHER

0–16 weeks

'My period was late, my breasts felt as though they'd been inflated with a bicycle pump. I felt sick, and on top of it all I felt utterly miserable.'

If that sounds like you, you are probably pregnant. For some women, the signs of pregnancy are crystal clear long before a pregnancy test confirms what you already know. For others, the symptoms are more subtle and, if you are not actually watching for them, it can be weeks or even months before the penny drops. These are the most common signs to watch out for.

1 *A missed period*, the sign we all know about but sometimes try to ignore. Some women continue to bleed at period times when they are pregnant, but it is usually much lighter than normal. The first missed period may coincide with the implantation of the fertilised egg and that can often cause blood spotting.

2 *Morning sickness*, which needn't happen in the morning at all. The majority of women feel some nausea though you won't necessarily be sick.

3 *Swollen and tender breasts*, which are even more tender than at period time. During a first pregnancy, nipples gradually darken in colour and little nobbles appear around the nipples. They are called 'Montgomery's tubercles'.

4 *Frequent peeing*

5 *Tiredness*

6 *Increased saliva*

7 *Food fads*

Getting a test

Even if you are certain you are pregnant, it is worth getting your knowledge confirmed. Your imagination can so easily play tricks on you, particularly if you are very keen to be pregnant, or very keen not to be. A pregnancy test will provide confirmation for most women, but beware of false negative results. A test will not usually show whether you are pregnant for two weeks after the expected date of your missed period (usually about six weeks after the last one). *You may get a positive result a few days earlier but an early negative result cannot be relied on. Wait a week, and do another one.*

Your urine (pee) will contain something called *human chorionic gonadotrophin* (HCG) if you are pregnant, this is why pregnancy tests are usually carried out by testing a sample of urine. Blood tests can also be done, at an even earlier stage of pregnancy, but they are expensive and not available everywhere.

It is best to collect a urine sample first thing in the morning, before you have anything to drink. (Any extra liquid will dilute the urine and make the HCG harder to see.) Put it in a clean bottle but make sure it contains no traces of detergent (it can change the result). Your GP should be able to test it for you at the surgery, or send it to the local hospital. Check how long the results will take. Some busy hospitals take up to a fortnight and some GPs these days are refusing to handle tests at all.

Your chemist may provide a pregnancy testing service, but it could cost as much as £5. You might be offered a do-it-yourself test. This may be cheaper but isn't as reliable. If it shows negative and you still don't get a period, try somewhere else.

The Family Planning Association or any family planning clinic can provide a test, free. *Women's centres* often provide a free, reliable, and friendly service. Look in your local paper or watch out for posters. *Pregnancy advisory services* are also reliable and cheap.

Seeing a doctor

If your result is negative, wait a week and do another. If it is positive or if you still get a negative result but feel that you may be pregnant, the best check is an internal vaginal examination by your doctor. He, or she, can tell by looking, and feeling, whether you are pregnant, even at this early stage. The neck of your womb may feel soft and your womb will feel bulky.

Some doctors still offer two tablets containing hormones as a way of testing pregnancy. If you are pregnant they will have no effect, if not, you will start to bleed. IF YOU ARE OFFERED THESE TABLETS, REFUSE THEM. The chemicals contained in them could, in rare cases, affect the development of your baby and they should never be prescribed for a pregnant woman. In fact if you think you may be pregnant avoid taking any drugs.

How does it grow?

To you it is still a missed period, but what is happening inside? Your baby started to develop as soon as egg and sperm made contact, high up in the fallopian tube. At first it was just a bunch of cells, dividing time after time to form an ever more complex organism. It took a week for this little cluster to find its way down the tube to the womb. Within the next three days it embedded itself in the wall of the womb. (Up to one in three pregnancies fail to get this far and miscarry as a heavy period.) Once safely embedded, the cluster feeds off the rich lining of the womb.

6 weeks   By the time your pregnancy can be confirmed by a test the cell cluster is about the size of a rice grain and the building of the brain, heart and digestive system is already under way. Medically you are now six weeks pregnant; doctors count from the first day of your last period (LMP).

8 weeks   Now the cluster is about the size of a peanut, looking rather like a monster from *Dr Who*, with a strange tail, eyes and the beginning of arms and legs.

12 weeks   The head is still quite large for the body, but the tiny clump of cells is now quite human in shape and about 2″ long. It moves and wriggles in a bag of amniotic fluid. By now the umbilical cord has grown, giving it a direct line to the placenta which provides its food and oxygen supply. This placenta grew out of the fertilised egg to provide a food bank, taking everything it needs from you, and filtering it through to the baby.

FEELINGS

'It wasn't until I was at least three months pregnant that I really believed it. I lay there thinking: "there's a baby inside me, and I'm going to have it."'

'I knew with absolute certainty that I was pregnant on the

*day I conceived. I was so certain that I ran around to my
friend's house to celebrate.'*

*'I really wanted this baby. We had planned it. I just
couldn't understand why I felt so unhappy.'*

These first weeks are a very mixed-up time. In a society which
makes it quite easy not to have children, choosing to have one
can take quite a lot of personal courage. The first pregnancy is
for most of us a step into the unknown. The world of children
and parents may be a totally alien one. A subsequent pregnancy
may raise other doubts: 'will I cope?', 'will the money stretch?'
'can I love another one as much?' A planned pregnancy may open
a Pandora's box of doubts and confusions about life and relationships. An unplanned one may be a crisis.

There is a sense in which every woman is alone in these
early weeks. The changes are happening to her body and, given
the world we live in, the greatest changes will happen to her life.
Jane remembered feeling very alone at this time:

*'I would lie there next to him but a glass cage had grown
round me. I didn't want to be touched, and yet I needed
comforting. I was crying out to talk about it, but I didn't know
what to say. His apparent lack of concern for the changes
taking place in my body made me want to scream with
frustration and rage. We had chosen this pregnancy together
but I was doing all the work of it on my own.'*

Her partner Mike didn't feel able to express his bottled-up feelings until the baby had been born. Then he said:

*'I wasn't ready for the sudden change. I couldn't see anything
different, but you had changed. You were much more
demanding. Nothing had happened to me at all so I couldn't
understand what was going on. There was nothing tangible.
You just felt rotten all the time. I was doing more housework,
coming home early to cook for you and yet I knew that you
didn't think I was doing enough so I felt both irritated and
guilty. I was worried and confused. I had to adjust to a new
relationship with you just as you had to adjust to the changes
in your body.'*

Fiona had recently ended a long relationship when she found
that she was pregnant:

'At first I intended to have an abortion. Then I started to think that, at 35, after two abortions, I was unlikely to get another chance. In the end, the main reason I had her was as a last connection with Don. Our relationship had lasted half my life. I knew that if I was ever going to have a baby, it would have to be his.

Most of the time I felt purposeful and businesslike about pregnancy but there were times when I felt very isolated and vulnerable.'

Even if you planned this pregnancy, you may be surprised to find that you are not as ecstatic as you expected to be. You may feel quite frightened at the step you have taken and find that others are impatient with you for needing so much reassurance and support. They cannot see your pregnancy and are unlikely to understand just what an emotional turmoil can be set off by the hormones racing around your body. It is a pity that more people don't realise how hard these early weeks can be. Most pregnant women feel both tired and sick at this time, and a tendency to weep may interfere with attempts at serious discussion, so it's not the best moment to be making an important decision. Nevertheless, if the pregnancy is accidental, a decision has to be made. If you are going to continue with the pregnancy you will want to banish the doubts as soon as you can and get on with planning your life. If it is going to end, the sooner it is done, the better.

Dealing with doubts

Talking to friends may help. You will probably find yourself going to the people most likely to confirm the decision you have already taken in the back of your mind.

The choice may seem quite extraordinarily hard to make and, if you continue with your pregnancy, you may find yourself plagued with doubts right until the end. Your confusion is not really surprising. There must be few people who can really feel 100 per cent certain about embarking on a journey they know so little about.

Talking to someone you don't know may be the most useful way of sorting your feelings out. Whatever you do, make sure it is what *you* want. Having a baby is too important for any of us to do as a favour for mother, husband or friend.

Deciding against

If you decide to end this pregnancy it need not be a decision against motherhood. There will be another opportunity. If it is a decision freely made you will not regret it either, but do act quickly.

Go first to your GP. Most will be quite sympathetic, and refer you to a local hospital. Unfortunately, in many areas of the country a combination of public spending cuts and lack of sympathy from senior doctors has made it almost impossible to get an abortion on the National Health Service. Ask your doctor what the position is in your area. If you are concerned about either your doctor's or the hospital's attitude, you will need to scrape together £100 and go either to the British Pregnancy Advisory Service (BPAS) or the Pregnancy Advisory Service (PAS). These services are non-profit-making charities set up to help women (see page 203).

Although you have made the decision alone, and will go through the operation alone, you will want, need and deserve to have someone to take care of you afterwards. You will probably feel physically fine, and very relieved, but you need to be allowed to grieve for what might have been.

HOW DO YOU GROW?

Quite astonishing things are happening to your body. Some lucky women sail through hardly noticing as their bodies change gear. Others find that every fluctuation causes a side effect. Knowing why you feel so strange might help you to cope with the feeling.

Nausea and fatigue are the twin miseries of early pregnancy. You may feel more tired than you have ever felt in your life. As it is often unexpected, the constant feeling of exhaustion can be one of the worst side effects.

Hormones are the culprits. During a normal menstrual cycle, the hormones progesterone and oestrogen rise, and then, if fertilisation does not occur, they fall again, causing a period to start. If you are pregnant the human chorionic gonodatrophin (HCG) builds up in your bloodstream. It nudges your ovaries into producing more progesterone and oestrogen. By the twelfth or fourteenth week the placenta has been formed in the womb to take over the job of supplying hormones and nourishment. As the HCG tails off and the placenta takes over, your symptoms may fade. If you have a pregnancy test after this time it may come back negative because the HCG may no longer show up in a urine test.

The best thing you can do is abandon your social life and get as much sleep as possible. If you have a rest room at work, take a packed lunch and make use of it. If not, try to find a corner where you can get your head down on a desk for a few minutes. If you are at home with a toddler it is even harder to get adequate rest. Friends may well help out to let you rest during the day.

Support from partners and friends really matters now. Housework on top of everything else may be more than you can stand. Off-load as much as you can. If you are alone, leave everything you can safely avoid, until you feel better.

For nausea, eat little and often, starting before you even get out of bed in the morning. Don't let your stomach get completely empty, or force yourself to eat salads now, they are not so easy to digest as the starchy foods. Potatoes and pasta may seem more appealing, and certainly help. Make sure you are well stocked with nutritious nibbles, and avoid greasy foods and alcohol. Vitamin B foods (wholemeal bread, wheatgerm, brewer's yeast) may be particularly helpful. At this time, let your stomach be your guide. If bread and butter is all you can manage (preferably wholemeal), eat it, it is far better than nothing at all. Nausea may be triggered by particular smells. Cooking may become a pretty miserable experience. Get your partner to do as much as possible or stick to the simplest things: bread, baked potates with cheese, fruit, yoghurt, porridge. Try to avoid getting overtired – it will make you feel much worse.

Though drugs are available against vomiting in early pregnancy, they are better avoided at this delicate stage of development unless the problem is so severe that you are losing weight and becoming dehydrated. If this does happen, and it is rare, your doctor will probably suggest taking you into hospital. Many women stop vomiting as soon as they get away from home, and rest. If you really cannot cope, try to get some time off, on your own and away from home. For nearly everyone the problem clears by the end of the third or fourth month.

Constipation is also caused by hormone changes. This time it is the progesterone, which slows down the action of, among other things, the bowels. Eat plenty of fibrous foods: fruit, vegetables and whole grain bread and cereals. You can add bran to most things – soups, stews or your morning cereal, if you need it. Be sure to drink plenty of liquids too. If you still find that you need a mild laxative, avoid liquid paraffin as it prevents the absorption of fat-soluble vitamins.

Frequent peeing occurs as soon as the uterus starts to grow and crowds out the bladder. It simply can't hold as much as it used to. As the womb rises out of the pelvic cavity after the first three months the problem will ease.

Contact lenses may suddenly feel uncomfortable because of the increased fluid in your body. As your eyes are largely liquid they will change in shape. If you have hard lenses you may well need to abandon them until your baby is born.

Vaginal discharge may increase, causing itching. You are also more susceptible to thrush (candida), a white discharge which is very irritating. Your doctor can prescribe pessaries for insertion in the vagina to cure the thrush, but as it may recur it is worth taking some preventive action: avoid wearing layers of tight clothing. Loose garments allow the air to circulate and cotton causes fewer problems than synthetics. Don't use scented soaps or vaginal sprays, but wash frequently with plain water. Adding vinegar to the bathwater helps guard against thrush by creating an environment in the vagina which discourages its growth.

Backache is unlikely to be a problem yet, but take care when you are bending and lifting. Your smooth muscle is softer than normal and an awkward movement could cause a painful 'slipped disc'. This is a good time to practise bending your knees and using your leg muscles to take the weight as you lift. Around the twelfth week, the joints between your pelvic bones, at the back, widen and separate. Occasionally they may pinch together on a nerve which runs down your leg, causing pain.

Insomnia frequently accompanies pregnancy. The pressure on your bladder may be to blame, it may simply be anxiety, or there may be no obvious cause. Everyone has a different recipe for curing insomnia. The main thing is to try and go to bed feeling relaxed. Don't wait until you are completely exhausted.

Dry, itchy skin can be a nuisance. Try adding a little milk to the water you wash in.

Food fads don't affect everyone, though most women find their sense of taste alters in pregnancy. You may find yourself craving for certain foods and turned off by others. Whether by accident or design, many women go off those things which are bad for them: alcohol, cigarettes, coffee, tea. What they crave may also turn out to be what they need, though it's hard to imagine how pickled gherkins could be an essential part of a diet!

Bleeding

There are several possible reasons for bleeding in early pregnancy. Until you have some idea why you are bleeding it is wise to lie down and rest. This is particularly important if you also have pain. Contact your doctor as soon as the bleeding starts and, even if it stops quite quickly, it is sensible to avoid sex for a couple of weeks.

Implantation bleeding happens when the egg attaches itself to your womb lining. So, if your last period was unusually light, it might not have been a period at all. Mention it to your doctor as it will make a difference to the estimated date for the birth (doctors will call it your expected date of confinement).

Bleeding at period times during pregnancy may be evidence that your body is not producing enough of the hormone progesterone. (This blood will be coming from the wall of the womb, not from the baby.) Once the production of progesterone has been taken over by the placenta at about three months, the bleeding will probably stop. Occasionally it continues into pregnancy.

If you have a history of miscarriage, you may be offered injections of progesterone to boost your supply. You must weigh this up very carefully. A hormone called Diethylstilboestrol, given to women in the 1950s, damaged some of the babies who were born. Some of those babies who have reached adulthood have been found to suffer from cancer and other abnormalities of the reproductive organs.

The hormone now used by doctors is a natural one which is said to be safer. Time will tell if the drug companies and doctors have got it right this time.

Bleeding after sex may just happen because a few fragile cells have been knocked at the neck of the womb. It isn't serious but it would be advisable to avoid sex (with penetration) for a couple of weeks.

Separation of the placenta is a common cause of bleeding after the first three months. The placenta, to which the baby is attached by the umbilical cord, may come away, or a little piece may break off. If the separation is slight, and the neck of the womb remains closed, the bleeding will stop.

A threatened abortion is the term used when you have the signs of a possible miscarriage (bleeding with pain in your tummy or lower back). You should contact your doctor and lie down until the bleeding stops. If it doesn't stop, and the pain continues, you may be surprised at how little your doctor has to offer, but by this time there is really nothing he or she could do to stop a miscarriage.

Miscarriage

Miscarriage is a shock, no matter how early it happens. You may feel grief, anger and real concern about your ability to have a baby. Friends often find it very hard to know what to say. They may make you feel even worse by saying cheerfully: 'It's all for the best really.' It is not likely that you feel that way and you have a right to feel sad. You may find another woman (or couple) who has been through this experience will provide a more sympathetic ear.

Doctors call an early miscarriage an 'inevitable abortion'. More than one in every ten pregnancies end this way. The most likely time is during the first three months – often so early that you won't even have realised that you were pregnant.

The reasons for miscarriage are not often clear. A very high proportion of early miscarriages are thought to happen because the baby was not developing normally. A virus, such as rubella, or an illness with a high temperature, may be a cause. Diseases such as diabetes, or a hormone deficiency (see *bleeding at period times*, above), can also be to blame, and you have a higher risk of miscarrying if you smoke, work with certain chemicals (see page 5) or have a very poor diet.

After the first three months, an 'incompetent cervix' may be suspected. This means that the neck of your womb (cervix) has been weakened (possibly by a previous birth, a womb scrape, or a number of abortions) and opens as the weight of the baby grows. In your next pregnancy a Shirodkar suture (a stitch) can be put in the cervix between the fourteenth and twentieth week to keep it closed.

It may also be that the placenta has failed to develop properly and is not providing enough nourishment for the baby. It is unlikely that exercise or sex, on its own, could cause a miscarriage. A baby that is healthy and well implanted is very hard to dislodge. It is sensible though to avoid both sex and strenuous exercise if you have already started bleeding.

The next time

'I wanted that girl so bad. I do everyone else's hair; I wanted my own little girl so I could do her hair and dress her up! When I look in the windows and see the little girls' clothes I just can't help myself – I have to run away.'

(from *When Pregnancy Fails*, by Susan Borg and Judith Lasker – see page 202)

The sadness of a miscarriage, particularly a late one, is not quickly forgotten. Eileen and John lost two babies, one at three months and a second traumatically at twenty-two weeks. The doctor told Eileen that she should spend five months of her next pregnancy in bed. She remembers the attitudes of her friends:

'They couldn't understand that to me it wasn't a choice. I wanted a baby so I had to go into hospital. Having been pregnant, I now felt even more strongly than before that I wanted to have a baby, whatever commitment it would take.'

There is no foolproof way of preventing a miscarriage, but it does seem to help to give your body a rest of about three months before trying again. If you rush into a second pregnancy you do run a slightly higher risk of a premature baby. You can use the space to make sure that you are in tip-top health: eat as well as you can, and get plenty of rest. From a psychological point of view you need time to get over the shock as well.

If you have only had one miscarriage, your chances of having a second one are no higher than they were before. If you have had two miscarriages you would probably do well to get advice from a doctor before embarking on a third pregnancy.

LOOKING AFTER YOURSELF AND THE BABY

It is not for nothing that a baby's birth weight is always recorded and announced after the birth. A healthy, bouncing baby is unlikely to suffer from the breathing difficulties and infections which so often affect low birth weight babies.

Of course, in these early weeks, you may feel too sick to eat very much (over 70 per cent of pregnant women feel this way). If you ate well before getting pregnant, your body will have the reserves to see you through these weeks. Catch up on good eating just as soon as you feel well enough.

Good eating

Here is a list to help you eat a balanced diet for pregnancy. Eat something from each group every day.

Vegetables   Two good helpings (at least) of fresh green, yellow or white vegetables.

Whole grains   A few slices of wholemeal bread or crispbread, a helping of whole breakfast cereal (see page 3), or a portion of brown rice or cracked wheat.

Fruit   At least one piece, preferably raw.

Dairy products   One to two pints of milk as a drink, in sauces, yoghurt, or cheese (¼lb of cheese = 1 pint of milk).

Meat, fish or eggs, or if you don't eat or cannot afford much meat, compensate by mixing pulses (cooked, dried beans) with grains or nuts, or by increasing the amount of dairy products you eat.

Drink as much as your thirst suggests but avoid sugary drinks which will spoil your appetite for good food. Stick to water, pure fruit juices, or herbal teas.

If you are still young enough to be growing yourself, if you are carrying twins, if you have had a baby, or a miscarriage, in the last year, or if you are still smoking or drinking, you should pay special attention to your diet. Read more about diet on pages 1–4.

Weight

A great deal of nonsense is talked about pregnancy and weight gain. The view used to be that every woman should 'eat for two'. Then everything changed about and pregnant women were led to believe that something dreadful would happen if they gained a little extra and that any extra weight would stay with them for ever. Now the pendulum is swinging back again.

A recent study in Minnesota, USA, indicates that underweight women are probably at greater risk than their overweight sisters of bearing low birth weight babies. A steady weight gain is perfectly normal. It is any sudden change, up or down, which should be mentioned to a midwife or doctor.

Most books suggest that in the first twelve weeks you will notice few changes in your body. Indeed some women actually lose weight now. Nicky and I gained weight straight away. We found our waists thickening within weeks of conception. We suspect that some other women do too, but that professional health workers rarely see, or weigh, them before the twelfth week and start their calculations from there. It might give you a clearer sense of your total weight gain if you do the same.

Recommendations for total weight gain vary enormously. One doctor, Gordon Bourne, who is clearly obsessed with the need for women to 'keep their figures', suggests that any gain over 8 or 9 kilos (18–20 lbs) will stay with you as fat. Our experience tells us a different story. We suggest that 9–13½ kilos (20–30 lbs) is about normal, gained at the rate of about ½lb per week in the first four months, doubling for the next three and then settling down and dropping off in the few days before birth.

You will not look like a sylph during your pregnancy, indeed why should you? You may only put on weight at the front, or you may seem to blow up all over. If you suffer from fluid retention, your doctor will want to keep an eye on that as your pregnancy progresses, but cutting down on food and fluid intake cannot make any difference and might do harm.

If you really are putting on weight at what seems to be an unreasonable rate, take a look at what you are eating. If you stick to the healthy diet we've outlined on pages 1 and 25, you shouldn't get fat. Cut down on sugary treats and substitute skim for whole milk but don't skimp the foods you need. You can do yourself and your baby more harm by eating too little of them than by eating too much.

Smoking and alcohol

Smoking is a difficult habit to break. Treat each day as a new start. It is never too late to cut down because the effect of smoking increases towards the end of pregnancy. If you cannot give up entirely try smoking only the first puffs and stubbing out the rest, or stopping a little earlier each evening. Alcohol can also affect the baby so try to limit yourself to an occasional drink and cut out spirits if you cannot manage to give it up entirely. Read about smoking and alcohol on page 6.

Drugs in pregnancy

Knowledge about the effect of drugs in pregnancy is limited. It is best to avoid any drugs which are not essential. For example, if you have a urinary infection you would be better to take antibiotics than risk a kidney infection but, if you have a cough or cold, try to cure it without drugs, and remember that even some vitamins are pretty potent. Don't take supplements unless you are sure you need them.

Here is a list of drugs which are suspected of causing problems in pregnancy. Remember that, even where there is a known link between the drug and birth defects, only a tiny number of babies will be affected.

In early pregnancy
Treatments for *epilepsy* and *cancer* have been associated with birth defects. You should get specialist advice if you are having treatment. **Warfarin**, used in blood clotting disorders, may cause abortions, stillbirth and birth defects. **Heparin** is a safer drug. **Anaesthetics** are also associated with miscarriage and there is some evidence that **corticosteroids** may cause problems but this is not confirmed. **Anti-thyroid** drugs and cough mixture containing **iodide** may affect the baby's thyroid which can lead to severe complications. **Minor tranquilisers** (such as **Valium**) and **codeine** (as a painkiller or in cough mixture) have both been associated with an increase in cleft palate. **Flagyl**, an antibiotic used in the treatment of trichomoniasis, has been shown to cause birth defects in animals though there are no similar findings with humans. **Tetracycline** may affect the baby's developing teeth. **Anti-nausea drugs** such as **Debendox** (now withdrawn by the manufacturers) have a suspected, but so far unproven, association with birth defects. **Oestrogens** and **progesterones** may affect the baby. **Stilboesterol**, an oestrogen used to prevent miscarriage in the 1950s, has been shown to lead

to cancer in some of the babies born. **Paracetamol** may be associated with kidney and liver defects though evidence is thin.

Vaccinations could damage the baby in early pregnancy.

In late pregnancy

Morphine and similarly addictive drugs may cause addiction in the baby; **epileptic drugs** can affect brain growth; **Beta Blocker** treatment for high blood pressure may affect growth and heart rate (**methyl dopa** has not been shown to cause similar problems); **minor tranquilisers** may make the baby limp and drowsy at birth and can cause a kind of colic which may last some time. **Lithium** may be associated with breathing difficulties (respiratory distress); and **aspirin** should be avoided in the final weeks as it can cause bleeding problems in labour.

THE PLACE OF BIRTH

Consider now where you want to have the baby, or you may end up with something you don't want. You have three choices:

1 A hospital birth under the care of hospital doctors and midwives;
2 A birth under the care of a midwife and your own doctor in a general practitioner unit (GPU) either in the local cottage hospital or a large hospital;
3 A home birth attended by community midwives and (usually) under the care of your own doctor.

Safety first

The established medical view in Britain is that no birth can be considered safe until it's over – that even among healthy women childbirth is not totally predictable, so therefore all births should take place in consultant units of hospitals. The less established view, based on similar evidence, is that technology, coupled with dangerously low staffing levels, creates more complications than it solves. So a healthy woman is safer giving birth at home, or at least in a GP unit with midwives in attendance, and the minimal technological interference.

Since opinions are so divided here, it's useful to look at how they do things in other countries.

Internationally

Holland and Sweden have the lowest rates of baby deaths (perinatal mortality as it is officially called) in the world, yet in Sweden virtually all babies are born in hospital while in Holland nearly 50 per cent are born at home. What these countries do have in common though are, firstly, highly trained and respected midwives who take charge of the whole process of normal pregnancy and birth, and secondly, social provision to ensure that nobody is too poor to eat well and take care of their health. The twin priorities seem to be midwife care and good basic health.

Here in Britain midwives are trained to care for women throughout pregnancy, labour and the early weeks of parenthood. Unfortunately they don't always get the chance to do so. Our maternity services are becoming doctor-dominated and this is not always to the advantage of women using the service.

Doctors are trained to cure the sick whereas midwives are taught to assist the healthy. The different approaches can have different consequences. When highly specialised doctors are in charge of childbirth they may be quicker to intervene with equipment and drugs. When midwives control services nature may have more of a chance.

Midwife antenatal clinics may also provide more continuity of care. The midwives running the clinic will see you regularly and know your individual pregnancy so they will be better able to make judgments about it than would a doctor who had seen you once in his life. But of course, individuals differ. Many women find that the most satisfactory antenatal care is given by their own doctors.

Keeping this information in mind, read the sections on place of birth and antenatal care before deciding what you want.

Hospital or home

Here is a comparative list showing the medical and social advantages of hospital or home birth.

Hospital	*Home*
1 Contact with other mothers can be very reassuring if this is your first baby.	1 You don't have to suffer separation from people you love. The experience will be shared.

2 Trained staff on tap can be a relief when everything is new.

2 You will have fewer professionals caring for you and less conflicting advice.

3 Domestic chores will not be added to difficulties of coping with a new baby.

3 Your sleep will not be disturbed by other people's babies.

4 Visiting will be regulated by the hospital. You won't be inundated.

4 Visiting can be regulated to your routines not the hospital's.

5 You have time to get to know your baby without pressures from other family members.

5 Your partner will be fully involved with the child from birth and probably more willing to share care.

6 Your labour can be followed electronically if you are at risk.

6 One person usually cares for you throughout labour. She is more likely to know you and, without technological equipment, may be more wary and spot problems before they get serious.

7 Modern equipment is available to deal with a crisis for you or your baby.

7 When high technology is not so conveniently at hand, unnecessary intervention is unlikely.

8 A special care baby unit may be available if your baby is in trouble.

8 Your baby will not be separated from you unless it is absolutely necessary.

9 Immediate treatment is available if your new baby should get ill.

9 A new baby is less likely to pick up a dangerous infection at home than in hospital.

Medical conditions indicating hospital birth
While a healthy woman with an uncomplicated pregnancy can make a personal choice about the place of birth, if you suffer from complications which may put you or the baby at risk you should probably book into a hospital consultant unit. Such conditions are:

General conditions   If you suffer from a chronic disease which needs regular medical attention you should discuss the matter carefully with your doctor. Diseases of the heart, kidneys or circulation, diabetes, epilepsy, tuberculosis, and other lung diseases can all create dangerous complications during pregnancy or birth. If you suffer from any of them you would be better off in hospital.

Drug or alcohol dependency can cause withdrawal symptoms in a new baby. Your baby would be safer where the early days can be medically supervised.

Herpes virus can infect a baby during birth. If you suffer from herpes (painful blisters which break out periodically around the genital area) and get an outbreak during late pregnancy you may need a Caesarean section (see page 101).

Previous birth problems which led to a Caesarean, high forceps delivery, severe post-partum haemorrhage (loss of blood) or retained placenta may recur so emergency equipment should be readily available.

Prematurity cannot be diagnosed in advance but if it has happened once you may feel safer booking your birth in a hospital which has facilities for vulnerable premature babies. Of course, if a home booked birth did start prematurely, you would automatically go into a hospital.

Unpredictable factors   Some conditions, such as twins, or pre-eclampsia, only appear later in pregnancy and will be discussed later. If complications occur a late hospital booking can always be made.

General risk categories
To be absolutely on the safe side you might like to know the factors which make home birth statistically more risky.
1 Age: if you are under 17 or over 35.
2 If you have already had four pregnancies. (Often the first is also considered more risky.)
3 If you are under 5ft 2in tall (see section on small pelvis, page 92).
4 If you are undernourished, overtired, a heavy smoker or in other ways not in good health.

Doctors will want to point out that, even if you do not come into any of these categories, there is no guarantee that your labour and the birth will be straightforward. If your baby's heart rate starts to fall you will not have the instant assistance which would be available in a consultant unit. Similarly, if you start to bleed very heavily, your own life could be at risk.

Most home birth advocates would rejoin that these problems

are far less likely to occur at home than in hospital in any case. The choice, in the end, must be yours.

ARRANGING A HOME BIRTH

As little as fifteen years ago, nearly one third of all births in Britain happened at home. By 1980 that figure had dropped to just over one birth in a hundred. It isn't that home births are more dangerous. On the contrary, better hygiene and heating have made home a safer place and, as we learn more about the process of labour, we should be better able to select those women who are least likely to run into problems.

Most doctors do not see things quite this way. Midwives may also be unhappy about home births. As the number drops, the midwives who used to deliver babies 'on the district' are getting rusty. They may be quite alarmed at being asked to revive these skills. Some women suffer little short of harassment in their attempt to give birth at home. One mother of three wrote a letter to AIMS (The Association for Improvements in Maternity Services) about the nightmares she had following a previous hospital birth. She said,

'I'm tired of being called irresponsible for exercising my right to have a baby at home. It is not compulsory to work in a factory, it should not be compulsory to give birth in one.'

If you really want to give birth at home, keep in mind at all times:
  1 **you have a legal right to give birth at home;**
  2 **you do not have to be attended by a doctor, a midwife is sufficient;**
  3 **the district health authority has a legal obligation to provide a midwife;**
  4 **it is illegal for an unqualified person to deliver a baby except in an emergency.**

Helping yourself
1 Speak to your own doctor. If he or she is willing to attend your birth you will be asked to sign a form EC 24 which is a contract

for care. Your midwife will be contacted by the doctor and will pay you a home visit to discuss arrangements.

2 If your doctor cannot attend try to find another who will. You do not need to leave your doctor's list for other services. Contact local childbirth groups, your community health council, other women or the organisations on page 203 for advice.

3 If no doctor is willing to take you on, you still have a legal right to be attended by a midwife. Write to the district nursing officer or nursing officer (community midwifery). One or other will be listed in the telephone directory under the name of your health district.

Your letter should include: (a) the date your baby is expected; (b) an explanation of your efforts to get medical cover; (c) a formal request for a midwife to be allocated to provide antenatal care and to deliver your baby at home; (d) the name of your doctor.

For your own safety you should find out whether the district midwives are equipped with oxygen and resuscitation equipment for the baby (including a laryngoscope, for clearing babies' tubes in case of breathing difficulties).

4 Some people simply hold out until labour is under way and then call a midwife. Of course she may then call an ambulance and admit you anyway. This option is not likely to lead to a relaxed birth which is the whole point of doing it at home. If you cannot get a midwife to co-operate happily you may be better off using your time to find the best hospital to give birth in.

Independent midwives practise in some areas. Many of these midwives set up independently just because they felt that the NHS was not supplying a sufficiently sympathetic and women-centred service. If you can afford a fee of £400–£500 (1983 figures), you can contact an independent midwife through a local birth centre, or via the Association of Radical Midwives (see page 203).

For emergency backup, make sure that there is an emergency obstetric unit (formerly known as the 'Flying Squad') operating in your area. An EOU is a team of qualified medical personnel who can get to you very quickly. Just dial '999' and ask for the emergency obstetric unit. Don't let anyone persuade you that you are asking for special privileges. These teams should be available everywhere to deal with obstetric emergencies. In fact the vast majority of visits are not for planned home births, but for emergencies in pregnancy.

Avoiding unnecessary intervention in hospital

It is harder to insist on doing things your way in someone else's place than in your own home. Nevertheless, many women simply feel safer in a hospital or, as one woman puts it,

'I felt that at home I would have been constantly worrying about the neighbours hearing me yelling. I had no idea whether I would need to yell, but I wanted to be somewhere sufficiently anonymous to yell in peace.'

You have a right to ask for referral to any hospital you like, provided they have room for you, though it's worth keeping in mind that travelling can be a nuisance both for check-ups and being visited afterwards and if your baby has to be kept in for any reason, a difficult journey can be a nightmare.

There is no substitute for local information. Talk to any other women you know and ask your doctor's advice. You can also contact local childbirth groups (see page 203 for addresses) or read the *New Good Birth Guide* by Sheila Kitzinger. You have three choices:

Consultant units are found in teaching hospitals, general hospitals and maternity hospitals. A consultant is a specialist, in this case a specialist in problem pregnancies and deliveries. If you have had a problem in your last pregnancy, or expect one in this, you will probably be very reassured by the medical approach and high-tech look of a consultant unit.

Many women whose pregnancies are quite normal will also be cared for in these units. Since the quality of care varies so much with individual consultants it is hard to generalise. In a few units you will find a great deal of encouragement for natural birth without drugs. In others you may find yourself subjected to much unnecessary routine.

Domino schemes can provide the best of both worlds. A district midwife comes to your home while you are in labour and then takes you into hospital, delivers your baby, and returns home with you six hours later. This has the advantage of hospital back-up and home comfort. Ask your doctor if a domino scheme operates in your area.

General practitioner units may be inside large hospitals (with all the emergency equipment a few seconds away), separate, or in a 'cottage hospital'. In a GPU you will usually be cared for by hospital midwives and your own doctor. These units are

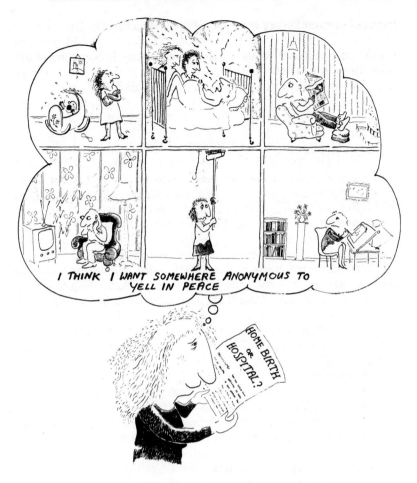

run by midwives for normal births and, though they are not always progressive in their methods of delivery and infant care, they are usually run on the understanding that nature should get first go before technology intervenes.

Check the record
Try and get hold of figures for various kinds of intervention and compare them to the national average. Don't forget that trends are changing all the time, usually for the better, so get recent figures if you can.

Induction (starting labour artificially) The national average rate is between 25 per cent and 36 per cent. Martin Richards, in the book *The Place of Birth*, estimates that a rate of 14 per cent would cover all medically necessary inductions. Some rates are now even lower than that.

Episiotomy (cutting the vaginal opening during delivery) is carried out routinely in some hospitals. The national average rate is 55 per cent (higher for first-time mothers). As recently as 1968 the rate was only 22 per cent. It is as low as 12 per cent in some hospitals and the rate in Holland is only 5 per cent.

Forceps In 1978 13.1 per cent of babies were delivered with forceps. The rate can be much higher; at Queen Charlotte's Hospital in London, for instance, the rate was 29.1 per cent in 1974. Recently the rate there has dropped a little.

Caesareans In 1982 10.6 per cent of babies were born by Caesarean section. This is a fairly low rate by international standards but it has risen by 29 per cent in four years.

Special care baby units Nationally, 15 per cent of newborn babies spend some time in special care. According to a 1974 study by Liston and Campbell, the rate was only 3.7 per cent when labour was spontaneous and between 12.9 per cent and 23.9 per cent for various forms of inductions. This could mean either that more 'at risk' babies are induced, or that induction puts more babies at risk.

Equipment isn't the only thing that can get in your way. Most hospitals now allow you to have your partner with you during labour but check these policies too:

1 Can your partner stay with you throughout labour and birth? (Some hospitals chuck them out when you need them most, e.g. during a forceps delivery.)

2 Can you bring someone as well as, or instead of, the baby's father?

3 Will you be allowed to move around during labour and choose your own position if the delivery is straightforward?

4 Will the baby be delivered on to your body? Will you be able to hold it and put it to the breast immediately after the birth?

5 Will the baby be with you in the ward afterwards, or in a nursery?

6 Will your other children be welcome to visit the postnatal ward and if so when, and for how long?

7 If you have any special dietary needs will they be catered for?

Who is who

You will be looked at by masses of different people during these months. They should all wear badges explaining who they are and giving their names. If you don't know who someone is or why they are talking to you then ask them. You are a healthy woman going through a normal experience and you have every right to know who is prodding your belly.

Midwives are not nurses, though most will have qualified as nurses before specialising in midwifery. They are trained to understand the process of normal pregnancy and labour. Student midwives usually wear white paper hats; qualified 'staff' midwives usually have a thick blue or purple line and senior 'sisters' wear frilly hats.

Doctors, when qualified, have authority over midwives and nurses even if they are less experienced. Student doctors will have *student* on their badges. They are unqualified. *House officers* are qualified but unspecialised. They will either have HO or SHO (senior house officer) on their badges. Then come registrars who are specialising in this area of medicine. They have *obstetric registrar* on their badges. *Consultants* are the top grade. They don't have their rank on their badges. You probably won't see much of your consultant even if his, or her, name appears on your card.

ANTENATAL CARE

'Doctors and consultants talk to the nurses about you as if you were a prize marrow, lying there on the couch. They should try talking to the patient, not behind her back,'

complained a Harrogate mother to her local community health council.

Antenatal clinics are often criticised for bad organisation and unhelpful treatment. Few of them provide any facilities for amusing other children and, as another mother in Harrogate told her community health council,

'going for a check-up was a complete afternoon of which your actual time spent with the consultant was approximately five minutes.'

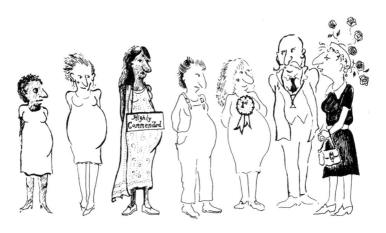

'I felt like a prize marrow.'

In spite of these difficulties, the vast majority of pregnant women attend the clinics regularly. In one study only 0.5 per cent of women booked into a large hospital had made fewer than two clinic visits and another study of 2000 women found only four non-attenders.

Clearly most women agree that antenatal checks are important. What they don't always know is how to make the best use of them. Again you have three choices:

Hospital clinics which, in spite of these reports, can be very well organised, cheerful places where you will meet other prospective mums and the staff who will care for you in labour. Some hospitals have organised their clinics at health centres which are much friendlier.

Your family doctor who can do all your antenatal checks provided he or she has done an obstetric training (a special course in pregnancy and childbirth). If your doctor has not done this training you can ask to be referred to another family doctor for antenatal care while remaining with your normal doctor for other treatment. (If your doctor cannot refer you, ask other mothers or contact the NCT or AIMS (see page 203) for suggestions.)

If your doctor works in a group practice or health centre your care may be mainly from district midwives working in the clinic. These may also be the midwives who deliver your baby if you have a home, or domino delivery.

Shared care means that your antenatal visits are split between your own doctor and the hospital. Most hospitals prefer to do at least the final checks if you are being admitted for delivery.

What are they looking for?

You will be expected to attend a hospital booking-in clinic, or have your first, full antenatal check at about twelve weeks. These checks are made to monitor your pregnancy for problems which might require more careful observation or treatment. You should go monthly for the first twenty-eight weeks, then fortnightly, and then weekly for the last month. The first visit provides a base line for measuring all future changes so it is important to go early in your pregnancy.

All the results of the tests carried out at these clinics will be entered in your notes and on your 'cooperation card' which you will carry with you if you are having shared care between your hospital and GP. An example of a 'coop card' is shown overleaf with explanation for all the shorthand terms used on it.

Routine tests

A mid-stream urine specimen (MSU)
This will be needed at this visit. You will be given two little pots with two pieces of cotton wool. The cotton wool is to wipe yourself with and the pot to pee in. You should collect, not the first drops of urine, but a 'mid-stream' sample which will then be analysed to ensure that you don't have an unnoticed infection of your kidneys (*asymptomatic bacteriaurea*). About one in every twelve or thirteen women have a kidney condition which they are unaware of. About half of them develop a more serious kidney infection during pregnancy which can cause complications, so it is important to check this early.

Urine tests
These are carried out on every visit so remember to bring a fresh sample with you each time (collected when you wake up). Make sure the bottle, which need only be a small one, is clean and well rinsed, as traces of detergent or jam could change the result. The urine will be tested for:

1 *Protein* The most common causes of positive urine tests are

YOUR COOP CARD EXPLAINED

On the front you may find the following initials:

Under Previous Pregnancies:
TDP, Termination of Pregnancy; LB - Live Birth, SB - Still Birth, PET - Pre-Eclamptic Toxaemia (see page 88); PPH - Post Partum Haemorrhage (see page 139).

This Pregnancy
LMP - last menstrual period; EDC (or EDD) - expected date of confinement (or delivery). WR/Kahn (or VDRL/TPHA) - these all mean the test for Syphilis. AFP - Alpha Feto Protein test (see page 68).

LONDON BOROUGH OF LEWISHAM
Health Department
PATIENT'S PERSONAL ANTE-NATAL RECORD CARD

Name (Block capitals—surname first): JONES JOANNA

National Health Service No.

Age: 27   Address: 83 The Avenue

Name of G.P.O. (Booked/not booked): Andrews   Tel. No. 6249
Address: 4 Sun Terrace Gdns

Name of G.P. (Booked/not booked): Peterson   Tel. No. 3911
Address: 29 St Davids Rd.

Name of Midwife   Tel. No.
Address

A.N Clinic: Oak Lane   Tel. No. 9676
Hospital (if booked): St. James   Tel. No. 2144

HISTORY OF PREVIOUS PREGNANCIES, MISCARRIAGES, LABOURS AND PUERPERIA

Year	Duration in weeks	L.B. or S.B.	Wt. of Baby lb. or oz.	A. or D. Age if	Duration of Breast Feeding	Pregnancy and Labour	Remarks Congenital abnormalities
1979	11	T.o.P.					
1980	40	L.B.	7. 11.	A	28 days	P.E.T. P.P.H	

Date of L.M.P.: 7/9/81   E.D.C.: 7/6/82

Investigations	Date	Result
W.R./Kahn	30/12/81	N.A.D.
Blood group		O
Rhesus		
Antibodies		

Chest X-ray

The patient is fit to have inhalation analgesia
(Signature of doctor)
(Date)

*IMPORTANT NOTE: In the event of a transfusion this record of the blood-grouping should always be checked and cross-matching should always be carried out.

M.C.W. 266

CONFINEMENT AND PUERPERIUM

Date of confinement ... Date discharged
Place of confinement
Notes on confinement

Puerperium

Mother's condition on discharge:
Breasts   Uterus
B.P   Perineum
Urine

Baby   Sex   Weight   Birth
Condition at birth   Discharge
Condition on discharge
Feeding

DATE FOR POST-NATAL EXAMINATION

POST-NATAL VISIT   Date
General condition

Duration of red lochia

Involution   Breasts
Weight   Urine   B.P   Hb
Vaginal examination

Feeding

Treatment or advice

Signature of doctor

When complete this card should be returned to the clinic stated on the front

E.G.&S.

In the Centre
Height of Fundus includes the estimated age of the baby (foetus) measured by dates, size, or US (sometimes USS) - Ultrasound Scan.
Foetal Heart this is judged by movements, MNF - movements not felt, or listening, H - heard, or FHH - foetal heart heard.
Presentation Br - Breech, C - Cephalic, Vx - Vertex, Eng - Engaged, NE - Not engaged, (all are explained on page 82).
BP, blood pressure (explained on page 44).
Oedema is explained on page 61.
Urine NAD - nothing abnormal discovered; Tr. Prot. - trace of protein; O Glucose - no glucose (see page 42).
HB haemoglobin, (explained on page 43).
Remarks Bloods - means blood tests done; Pregaday - iron tablets; Mat BI - maternity grant claim form; Vag Disch - vaginal discharge (pessaries given); 3/7 in three days; Oestriol (see page 99); wt. - weight; wt ↑ - weight up; wt ↓ - weight down.

First Examination: Date ? 12.81
Height 5'3"   Nutrition ✓   Bowels ✓
Teeth ......   Arrangements for dental treatment ......
Estimation of pelvic capacity ......

Breast ✓ wants to breast feed
Heart ...... N.A.D
Lungs ...... N.A.D
Varicose veins ......
Date of quickening ? 20.1.82

Date	Height of fundus (weeks)	Presentation and Position	Foetal Heart	B.P.	Oedema	Urine	Weight st. lb.	Hb.	Remarks and advice given, treatment, drugs, mother-cntr classes, etc.	Next Appointment Initials Dr. or M/W
7.12.81	dates/ 5.35 12/15	—	MNF	120/75	—	NAD	9-3		Wants shared care + early discharge	BJ → hosp.
30.12.81	16	—	—	130/85	—	NAD	58	12.3	U/S Bloods → GP	32 wks
5.2.82	20/22	—	FHF 4/52	99/60	0	Tr. Prot. o.gluc	10-0 63.5		Pregaday	BJ 4
5.3.82	dates 27 U/S 26	F 26 Br	++	95/60	—	NAD	10-6		U/S on 10.1.82 = 18 weeks single. EDD 8.6.82 ✓ Mat BI	BJ 3
19.3.82	U/S 24/28	Br	++	95/60	—	NAD	10-8		See at 32 weeks - hosp.	
16.4.82	32	C	FHHR	100/65			69	10.9	Check Hb	
30.4.82	34	Vx	++	110/60	ankle +	NAD	11-0		Vag. disch. Pessaries. Double iron. Watch weight	
14.5.82	36	C NE	++	125/95	finger + ankle +	Tr. Prot.	71.0		Rest + check BP + urine 3/7 Oestriol + U/S	
17.5.82	37	C	++	130/90	+	NAD	71.0		See 3/7	
21.5.82	38	C	++	140/90	+	Tr. Prot.	10.5		Admit for rest weight static	
4.6.82	39 by U/S	Vx NE		120/80	sl.		11-0		In hosp. for rest 3/7 wt. static ∴ hosp. next week.	
11.6.82	T	C		130/90	+		70		Wt ↓ Admit for induction Tues	

contamination from a jar that wasn't completely clean and vaginal discharge; but if protein is found you will be asked to do a mid-stream specimen just to check that you don't have an infection. In later pregnancy, protein can indicate that you have pre-eclampsia, a serious condition needing hospital admission (see page 88).

2 *Glucose* Over 50 per cent of women have a raised glucose level in their urine during pregnancy. A positive test may be caused by sweets (it's worth mentioning if you have just eaten some), because in pregnancy sugar is more likely to spill into the urine. This is not a problem. It could also indicate diabetes. Diabetes can be triggered by pregnancy and, though it would probably clear up once the pregnancy is over, it is likely to return during subsequent pregnancies and get worse.

(A *glucose tolerance test* can establish whether you have got diabetes. You are given glucose to drink and then a series of blood and urine tests will be taken over a period of time to check whether the level of sugar drops, or stays high, which is an indication of diabetes. If you do have diabetes, you will be referred for specialist help in controlling your condition through diet; if necessary you will also be given insulin, and you should certainly give birth in hospital.)

3 *Ketones* These are evidence that you are eating so little that your body is breaking down fats for energy. This is most unlikely to occur in early pregnancy unless you are vomiting very severely.

Blood tests
Blood tests taken from a single blood sample will be carried out at your first visit, and then again towards the end of your pregnancy, and after the birth. The tests are looking for:

1 *Your blood group*, in case of the unlikely event that you will need an emergency blood transfusion. If your blood group is RH negative you will need a shot of 'Anti-D' after the pregnancy. This is because a RH negative mother, carrying a baby with a different blood group, may build up 'antibodies' to protect her own bloodstream against the baby's blood. In the first pregnancy, both mother and baby will be unaffected by the different blood groups, but if the Anti-D injection is not given the build up of anti-bodies may endanger future babies during pregnancy.

2 *RH antibodies*, which may have built up if you were not given Anti-D after a previous birth, abortion or miscarriage. In

this case your pregnancy will need very careful monitoring and you will probably be referred to a hospital specialising in this condition.

3 *Anaemia* This *haemoglobin* test is a measurement of the proportion of oxygen carrying pigment in the red blood cells in the blood plasma. A normal measurement lies between 12 and 14. During pregnancy, the number may drop to 10, without any problems. If it drops below that figure you should take the iron and folic acid supplements offered which should increase the haemoglobin in the red blood cells which carry oxygen to the baby.

You may not need these supplements at all so wait for the blood test results before taking them. Some doctors believe that anaemia in pregnancy is much rarer than it seems. They say that the number of red blood cells seems low only because there is a much greater volume of blood during pregnancy. Others see the low levels as evidence of anaemia requiring iron treatment. Most clinics just give iron to everyone.

If your haemoglobin level was normal at the start of pregnancy, you may decide against taking iron supplements, particularly if they make you feel more nauseous and constipated (as they sometimes do). However, if you are not taking supplements, make sure you eat plenty of food containing iron: dried beans, beansprouts, prunes, liver, green vegetables, eggs, meat and brewer's yeast; Eat foods containing folic acid (green leafy vegetables) and vitamin C (mainly in fruit). Iron cannot be properly used by the body without these other foods.

If your haemoglobin level drops, you would be sensible to take supplements of iron and folic acid. Adequate iron stores will stop you from getting run down and give you some back-up if you should happen to bleed heavily during labour.

If the brand of iron you are getting makes you feel ill, ask for a different kind – they don't all have the same effect.

4 *Syphilis*, hepatitis B, or any other infectious conditions which could be harmful to you and the baby. (Hepatitis B is highly contagious. Medical staff will wear gloves for all examinations if you are a carrier.)

5 *Rubella antibodies* which will be found if you have been immunised against German measles or have had the disease. If you haven't got any antibodies you will be immunised after the birth just to make sure that you don't contract German measles during another pregnancy as this would be dangerous for the

baby. (You may be offered Depo-Provera, the injectable contra-ceptive, at the same time. Don't accept it. The manufacturers now agree that this drug should not be given in the period im-mediately after a baby is born (see page 177).)

If you are in contact with rubella during pregnancy you should contact your doctor for blood tests even if you have been immunised. Occasionally the immunisation doesn't work.

6 *Sickle cell and thalassaemia,* conditions of the blood which may be passed on to the baby and may, in themselves, put both mother and baby at risk during pregnancy.

Sickle cell trait is a condition which affects some one in ten of all Asian, Arab and black people, and occasionally Mediter-ranean people as well. The 'trait' is not in itself a problem, but if it comes up on the test, you may want to find out if your partner has it too, which would increase the chances of passing '*sickle cell disease*' on to the baby.

Sickle cell disease and *thalassaemia* are rather more serious. They are both forms of anaemia which would require careful monitoring during pregnancy. Extra folic acid would be pre-scribed and, in the case of sickle cell, blood transfusions may be necessary, though both conditions can strike in a fairly mild form.

There has been a lot of criticism from the black community about the lack of research into these diseases. If you want more information contact The Sickle Cell Society (see page 204).

7 *A folic acid deficiency* test will be done if you are anaemic. If you are deficient you will be given folic acid supplements. In many hospitals now folic acid is automatically given with iron tablets. According to Adele Davis, the American nutrition writer, one-third of all pregnant women are deficient in this vitamin. She feels that lack of vitamin B6 (pyriodoxine) may also be to blame for anaemia. These vitamins occur in green leafy veg-etables and in whole grains and yeast which are also good sources of iron.

Your blood pressure

This will be checked at every visit. You cannot feel changes in blood pressure, but they could be an early warning sign of pre-eclampsia (see page 88). Your blood pressure (BP) is a measure-ment of the pressure at which your heart is pumping blood through your body. If your heart starts pumping faster, the blood vessels become narrower, or your blood gets too thick, the BP will rise.

It is recorded as two numbers written on top of each other like fractions. The top number is the systolic, when the heart is pumping, and the second is the diastolic, when it is resting. Neither of these numbers should change much during pregnancy, though rather more concern will be shown if the diastolic (the lower number) starts to rise.

The actual numbers vary from one person to another, but generally the lower number shouldn't rise by more than 15 to 20 or go above 90. Some women will have a BP of 140/90 or more at the start of pregnancy. This means they have 'essential' high blood pressure and the pregnancy should be monitored by a specialist.

Weighing and measuring

A weight check is done each time so try to wear similar weight clothes. You are being monitored in case you gain weight suddenly, which can be a symptom of pre-eclampsia, or you are not gaining enough, which could indicate other problems. Don't be intimidated into dieting strictly to keep your weight down. (See page 25 on weight.)

Your height will be recorded and the midwife will note any signs of physical abnormalities which could affect the size and shape of your pelvis. You may be asked your shoe size – someone with small feet may have a small pelvis. (On the other hand, one of us has small feet and an enormous pelvis.)

History taking

At this visit you will be taken aside by a midwife for a discussion of your medical and social 'history'. The information requested is necessary to the careful monitoring of your pregnancy even though the questions asked may not appear to be. Many of these questions will also be asked about your husband. Some hospitals seem embarrassed to make enquiries about your partner if you are not married, but the information is no less important, so, if you know it, pass it on.

1 *Personal details* Your name, age, race, country of origin, religion, occupation and marital status. Some questions may appear offensive, but bear in mind that, if your mother came from Jamaica, or your father from Greece, you could have sickle cell or thalassaemia. The technician doing the blood checks can-

not actually see you, but the note with the sample will ensure that these checks are made. Give full information about your work so that the medical staff will know whether it could affect your pregnancy.

2 *Family history* of diseases or conditions which could be passed on such as twins.

3 *General medical history* including past or present diseases and allergies.

4 *Surgical history* of any operations, blood transfusions, serious accidents.

5 *Contraception* previously used is recorded, or if you have been infertile for any length of time, that will also be noted.

6 *Menstrual history*, the age you started, the normal length of time between periods, their regularity and the day of your last period are all noted.

Your delivery date should be nine calendar months and one week after the first day of your last period. If you normally have a long cycle (thirty-five days), add an extra week to your calculation, if it's a short cycle (twenty-one days), subtract a week, but remember, this is just a guide, two weeks either side of the date is just as likely.

7 *Your last pregnancies* will give clues about this one so give details of any problems you experienced. Similarly, give details of your previous labours, and your own and the babies' health afterwards, including previous babies who have been adopted, and abortions (TOPs). Since about one in every four women are likely to have had abortions, don't be embarrassed to mention them. If for any reason you don't want an abortion or adoption recorded on your notes, say so.

If you were unhappy about your treatment during a previous pregnancy or labour, now is the time to say what happened, explain any fears you have, and ask for assurances that this time things will be better.

Ask your questions now, you may not get another chance (see pages 35–6). Some midwives are quite hostile to these questions. They feel hurt and angry about criticism levelled at the health service by consumer groups over the past few years and they are inclined to react very defensively. Keep this in mind and put your demands tactfully and politely as well as firmly. After all it is better to have your midwife on your side when you are feeling vulnerable during labour.

Pain relief may be discussed so read the section on page 125 to prepare yourself.

Physical examination

You will now see a doctor for a full physical examination for which you will be asked to undress completely.

Your teeth, breasts, nipples, heart and lungs will all be checked to see that you are in good physical shape and need no special monitoring.

Then the doctor will put a hand on your tummy to find the top of your uterus (*height of the fundus*). The bump will gradually move up as your pregnancy progresses, giving a fairly reliable guide to your delivery date and length of pregnancy. Then she (or he) will put the other hand inside the vagina and feel the bulk of the uterus between her hands. At the same time you will be checked for any pelvic abnormalities and a smear test may be done for analysis.

This examination is the most thorough one you will get; further routine visits will require only a hand on your tummy, a few questions and no internals until late in pregnancy.

YOUR RIGHTS AT WORK

Unfair dismissal

The Employment Protection Act (1974) gives you some protection against dismissal during pregnancy, provided,

you have been in your job at least one year, or two years if your boss employs fewer than twenty people, or, five years if you work less than sixteen hours per week (and more than eight).

If you qualify, your employer cannot legally dismiss you unless:

you are incapable of doing the work, or it would be illegal for you to do the work, and he is unable to find you safe alternative work.

If your employer has the right to dismiss you for these reasons, you will not lose your rights to maternity pay and job reinstate-

*ment after the birth, provided you qualify for them (see page 72).
If you resign you will lose the lot.* If you believe you have been
unfairly dismissed, you have three months in which to make a
complaint to a tribunal. Get form IT1 from your job centre or
employment office.

Time off

Paid time off for antenatal care is your legal right according to
the 1980 Employment Act, no matter how long you have had
your job or what hours you work. After the first visit you may be
asked to provide an appointment card as evidence that you really
are going to the clinic. This is an ideal opportunity to discuss any
possible risks of your working environment with your doctor, and
ask him or her to notify your employer of any special arrangements which may be necessary to protect your health.

Coping at work

*'I didn't tell anyone until I was about five and a half months
pregnant and I think that was a mistake. If everyone knows
you are pregnant, even if you don't look like it, it is easier to
get away with being grumpy and sick. I certainly should have
rested more but as no one knew I needed to I couldn't justify
it.'*

There is something special about being pregnant and your work-
mates, and even your employer, will probably respond sympath-
etically to your needs if you let them. Of course you are not ill,
and may well feel absolutely wonderful, but if, like Sara, quoted
above, you feel grim, it's fairer on both you and them to say what
you need, accept your shortcomings and be grateful for offers of
help: the comfortable chair, an extra hand to shift a typewriter,
the chance to put your feet up while someone else brings your
lunch. (Of course, if you haven't been in your job for a year you
might prefer to keep quiet in case of dismissal.)

Hazards at work

Once you are pregnant, you do have some protection under the
law against chemicals or working practices which might be
harmful (see section on rights at work, page 5).

Such hazards may include heavy lifting, working with dangerous chemicals and excessive stress. If you are concerned about substances at work, show the lists on pages 5–6 to your union health and safety representative and ask for his, or her, help in finding out whether you are exposed to any of them. If there is no union where you work, discuss the matter with your doctor and ask for a letter to your boss requesting information about possible toxic substances, or suggesting that you should be moved to a safer job during your pregnancy, if there is evidence that you may be at risk.

Health at work

Unless you are working with chemicals, you should not need a change of job in early pregnancy. However, if you suffer from nausea, which is worse if you are tired, you may find that an extra break to put your feet up will be readily accepted by your employer, or at least overlooked:

'We could take a break when we wanted because our overseer was based in another department and we were left to ourselves.'

Or you may not be so lucky:

'We can only use the rest room during the dinner hour. My blood count was very low so I'd fall asleep during my work and there was nowhere I could go. If I wanted to rest I'd go to the toilet. If I was really tired I'd fall asleep on the toilet.'

(Quotes from *Pregnant at Work*, Sue Rodwell and Liz Smart, Open University, 1982).

If you are not given due consideration during pregnancy, take the matter up with your trade union or personnel department.

A suggested code of practice for trade unions and employers

* Ensure that employees are informed of their statutory and negotiated rights.
* Check that pregnant employees are not working with sub-

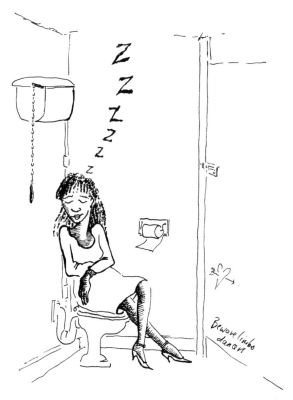

Not all work-places provide adequate rest-rooms

stances which could be harmful to their babies and arrange alternative work if they are.
* Allow short breaks for snacks if an employee in early pregnancy suffers from nausea.
* Ensure that pregnant employees have access to the rest room (if available) throughout the day.
* Where possible arrange flexible work times to avoid rush hour travel when an employee requests it. (In an Islington community health council survey, rush hour travel was mentioned as a major difficulty.)

* Ensure that employees are not unreasonably denied time off for antenatal checks.
* Ensure that canteen food is nourishing and that fresh fruit, fruit juices and milk are regularly on sale.
* Ensure that pregnant employees are not expected to do arduous work or heavy lifting particularly in late pregnancy.

OTHER RIGHTS AND BENEFITS

Free prescriptions and dental care are yours by right during pregnancy and the first year after the birth. A form, FW8, should be available at your local clinic or can be picked up at the social security office. It must be signed by a doctor or midwife. Once it has been sent off, you are entitled to sign the back of any NHS prescription form, and you will be excused payment. The dentist will also ask you to sign a special form.

Free milk and vitamins are available if you have two children under 5 years old (apply on the same form, FW8, as above). If you have a low income fill in a form MV11 from any social security office and you may also qualify. Pregnant women on supplementary benefit or family income supplement qualify automatically. The allowance is seven pints of milk per week and two bottles of vitamins every three months.

Fares to the clinic can be claimed if you are on family income supplement or supplementary benefit just by showing your order book to the hospital social worker. If you are on a low income the hospital can give you another form, H11, to fill in and send to the social security office for a refund.

Chapter 3

THE RETURN OF SANITY

16–28 weeks

'He had already fallen asleep when I felt it, a little tickle, a flutter, inside. I lay very quiet to see if it would happen again and it did. I was enormously excited and woke him up shouting, "I felt the baby move" – then it stopped and he couldn't feel a thing. But it was wonderful. That little thing inside was knocking on the wall to let me know it was there. For the first time, I felt there was someone there, someone separate from me.'

How does it grow?

16 weeks   It is still pretty strange-looking, small enough to fit in the palm of your hand and covered with fine down. The eyes and mouth seem to take up far too much space on its face. If you have already been pregnant before you may be able to detect movements as early as this, occasionally even earlier, but they will be very faint.

Your baby's heartbeat can now be heard with a Sonicaid or Doptone. This little instrument, laid on your tummy, amplifies the sound so you can hear it too.

20 weeks   By now you will probably have felt your baby move. Some people describe it as like 'a little fish' or a butterfly. At first you may mistake the feeling for indigestion or a tummy rumble but you will soon realise that it is quite independent of you.

The baby has reached half its birth length, though it still weighs only about half a pound. Hair has started to grow but the heart, brain and respiratory system still need refinement.

24 weeks   Just over twelve inches from top to toe, your baby is now quite well-formed, but rather skinny. A white, vaseline-like substance now covers the body to protect it against

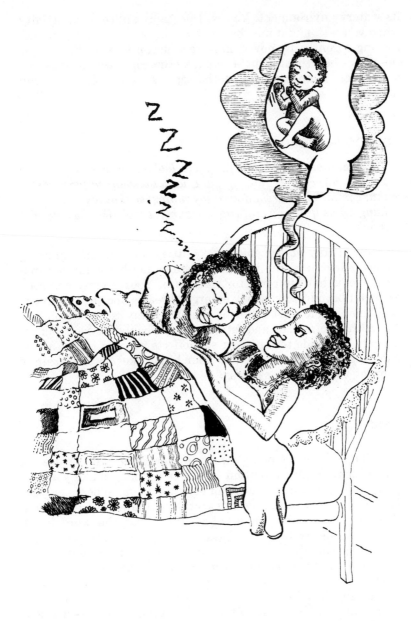

'He had fallen asleep when I felt a little tickle . . . a flutter . . . that little thing was knocking on the wall to let me know it was there.'

its watery environment. You will probably notice most activity when you rest, and it may be quiet when you are moving around, rocking it gently. By now a midwife or doctor will be able to hear the baby's heartbeat using a 'foetal stethoscope', which looks like a trumpet. If an ordinary stethoscope is used, ask if you can listen too.

HOW DO YOU GROW?

'I feel fat, not fruitful, just fat, I was looking forward to looking curved and glowing but I hadn't bargained for breasts that completely overshadowed my tummy so that my clothes hang off as if from a cliff edge. Frankly, I look like the side of a bus.'

Of course many women enjoy every little change in their growing bodies. For others, the in-between stage, neither sylph nor matron, seems hard to come to terms with. Your tummy will soon grow out beyond your newly enlarged breasts and then everyone will know you are not suffering from too many second helpings!

Although nausea and fatigue will probably lift soon, here is a top-to-toe guide to the other side effects you can expect as the baby takes up more room, and your body takes on the strain of running two separate systems.

Head

Face   Some women glow during pregnancy but we are not all so lucky. Water retention (see page 61) may make you look puffy and sometimes a 'mask' of dark colouring appears on your face. If you find the mask embarrassing, make-up will cover it though you may be comforted to know that the word for it, chloasma, means the special tint of a growing shoot or bud. It will disappear after your pregnancy. According to Adele Davis, nutrition writer, extra folic acid (found in green vegetables) will help.

Nose   Bleeding is a common problem due both to the increase in your blood supply and to the effect of the hormone progesterone which makes the walls of your blood vessels softer. The hormone effect may also give you a *runny nose* as the membranes of your nose are also softer and less efficient. Both problems will go after the birth.

Teeth   There is an old saying that a woman loses a tooth for every baby. In fact the *calcium* which your baby needs for its bone formation will be taken from your bones which is why it is important to keep eating calcium-rich foods to replace it (see page 60).

Gums are more of a problem. You may find that they get quite sore and bleed easily when you brush your teeth. This is that hormone progesterone at work again making them soft and spongy and prone to an infection called gingivitis. Your gums need to be treated properly or they may start to recede exposing the roots of your teeth. If this happens your teeth will be more likely to decay and, if the gums recede far enough, may actually drop out.

Dental treatment is free during pregnancy. Ask to have your teeth cleaned, and get the plaque removed. The best way to prevent gum problems is to eat chewy whole foods and raw vegetables as well as massaging your gums with a soft brush every time you clean them. If at first they hurt too much, get a toothpaste specially for sensitive teeth, such as Sensodyne, which will take the pain away enough for you to brush them properly.

Breasts

Breasts may be quite painful. Some women find it almost impossible to be touched, even gently, while others find the extra sensitivity sexually stimulating. Towards the middle of pregnancy, the extreme sensitivity should disappear.

Your breasts will grow considerably in size. Some women enjoy this busty look, others loathe it. By the sixteenth week, you are already able to produce milk. You may find that a yellowish substance called colostrum will come out if you squeeze your breasts just above the nipple. Your baby will drink it for the first few days before your milk comes in. If you can't easily squeeze any out, don't worry, your baby won't have the same problems.

Nipples sometimes cause concern. Are they too big, flat, of the wrong shape? In fact, a hungry baby can latch on to almost any shape, but if yours turn inwards (like a dimple) you could try persuading them to turn the other way. Very gently draw them out with your fingers. Your partner can do it for you and you will find that gentle sucking has the same effect. Some women wear *Woolwich Shells* under a bra to coax them out. They are made of glass, and can be bought in a chemist or at the clinic. In fact nipples which appear to be a difficult shape at the start of pregnancy, often change before the birth.

Some clinics advise you to rub cream into your nipples to prepare them for breastfeeding. There is no evidence that this helps.

Bras are not compulsory during pregnancy, but if your breasts are very heavy, they may be more comfortable. You will probably need at least two sizes larger than you usually wear, but try some on. Look for wide straps. If your bras are also made of cotton, and front opening, they may be suitable to wear while breastfeeding. It is better to buy them with cups slightly on the baggy side and without stitching on the cups so that they don't rub on tender nipples.

Although many people say that wearing a bra avoids stretch marks, there is actually no evidence of this.

Tummy

A dark line, the *linea nigra*, may appear down the middle of your tummy. It will fade after the birth.

Your stomach should be having a well-earned rest during these middle months though you may still find that there are some foods which you cannot eat. If you are unlucky *heartburn* and *indigestion* may start early. Heartburn is caused by the acid contents of your stomach backing up into your throat. It happens because the muscles, which usually keep the entrance to your throat closed, are slacker than usual.

Eat little and often and prop yourself up on pillows at night to encourage the contents of your stomach to stay down. Don't take sodium-based indigestion remedies such as Alka Seltzer or baking powder which will make you blow up with wind. Antacids such as Rennies or Settlers may give temporary relief. Mint tea can be a comfort. Add two teaspoons to a pint of boiling water, and drink it after meals.

Make sure that your evening meal is digestible and don't eat too late. Chewy foods are better kept for earlier in the day and should be very well chewed.

Constipation can be a problem throughout pregnancy so keep eating plenty of high fibre foods. You can put extra bran in your morning cereal if salads give you indigestion. Remember to drink plenty of water too.

Pains in the stomach or anywhere below the navel should be reported. You may well have strained a ligament under your belly, which is not cause for concern, but pains could indicate something more serious.

Your cervix (the neck of your womb) may grow a layer of fragile cells which are easily damaged during sex. You will only notice this 'erosion' as it is called if you get slight spotting after making love. Little growths called polyps, can also grow in the cervix. They are also quite harmless but may cause spotting after intercourse, or an internal examination.

Bottom

Haemorrhoids (piles) are varicose veins of the anus. They can be very painful and fear of the pain can stop you going to the toilet which may lead to constipation and make things worse. The doctor or clinic may prescribe cream to ease the pain and shrink the piles. Get treatment early, they don't go away by themselves, though you could try one home remedy: a peeled garlic clove pushed up at night. Some people find it very effective.

If the piles are sticking out, you can try, very gently, pushing them back in while sitting in a bath (that softens them). You should then push them back each time you go to the toilet. If you cannot manage while you have piles without a laxative, avoid liquid paraffin which interferes with vitamin absorption (see section on constipation, above).

Peeing constantly will be less of a problem as your womb rises out of the pelvis giving your bladder a little more room. You may still suffer from *cystitis*, an infection of the bladder and urethra (the tube your pee travels through), which makes it burn. If you do, stick to loose clothing; avoid nylon or other synthetic knickers or tights; always pee before and after making love; and empty your bladder as soon as you feel the urge, don't hang on. If you do feel the slight itching which heralds a cystitis attack, drink as much water as you can, the liquid may flush the bacteria out of your system before an infection takes hold. If not, see your doctor for treatment.

Back

Backache should always be reported to the doctor in case you have a kidney infection (see page 39). Your back will also be taking a lot of extra strain and you should protect it by learning to use it properly. The illustration on page 59 shows you best how to bend and carry. Give piggy backs rather than hip rides to your toddler and, when getting out of bed, roll on to your side, don't just sit straight up.

Exercises can help an aching back (see picture). (You can do a similar exercise lying flat on your back and then arching and flattening it against the floor). Avoid exercises which strain your back and tummy muscles such as sit-ups and leg lifting and do your exercises slowly. You want to stretch your muscles, not pull them. In fact the best overall exercises you can do are swimming or yoga which gently stretch everything.

Vagina

Varicose veins of the vulva (the entrance of the vagina) can be another misery. The pain can best be relieved by the use of a pad held tightly against the vein on a sanitary belt. (Vaginal itching and discharge have already been mentioned on page 21).

Pelvic floor muscles are the ones which form a ring around the vagina. They will be stretched to the limit during labour. If you have toned them up (see page 8) and kept them supple they should snap back quite quickly. If not they may go saggy like an old bra elastic.

Vaginal bleeding is not uncommon in pregnancy but should be taken seriously. Inform your doctor and then lie down until the bleeding stops. If it continues, or gets worse, keep your doctor informed or contact the maternity unit at your nearest hospital. (For more about bleeding look back to page 22.)

Legs

Your thighs will thicken as well as your belly because your body needs to lay down extra fat to see you through the early days of breastfeeding.

Cramps in your legs may occur, especially at night. If you

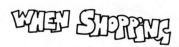

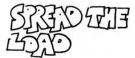

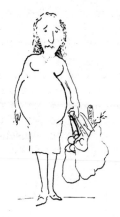

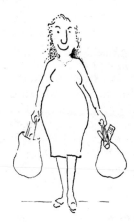

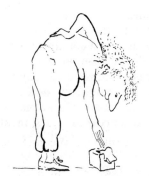

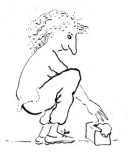

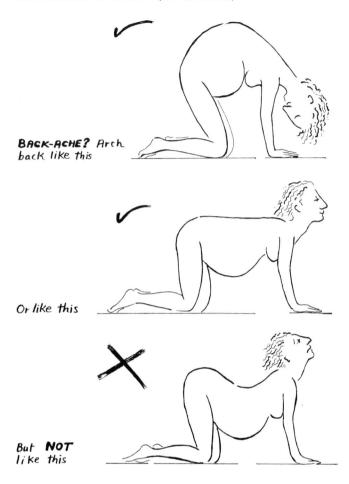

BACK-ACHE? Arch back like this

Or like this

But **NOT** like this

are woken by a cramp (you can't miss it, an acute, sharp pain), grab your toes and pull them sharply towards you while forcing your heel up. Alternatively, stand on the floor and push your heel down hard. Then massaging helps to ease the pain away.

It isn't clear why some people get cramps but it may be that you are lacking in salt or calcium. You could try eating something salty in the evening before going to bed and make sure that your diet is rich in calcium. Good sources are nuts, meat and milk products. You can take calcium tablets as well if necessary. (check with your doctor for the dose). Since calcium is not easily absorbed without vitamin D, some milk products or fish should also be eaten. Avoid adding chocolate to your milk, as it prevents calcium absorption.

Varicose veins may cause your legs to ache. The extra blood volume combined with softer blood vessels makes you more prone than usual to varicose veins. If you already have them they may get worse. Wearing support tights will be a great help. (You can get support stockings on prescription.) Put them on before you get out of bed in the morning so that the extra support for your blood vessel walls is there as soon as you stand and put a strain on them. If you find that inconvenient, rest with your legs horizontal for a few minutes at least, before putting them on. Try to put your legs up (on another chair if necessary) as often as you can during the day. If they are aching at the end of the day lie down if you possibly can.

All over

Water retention (oedema) may make your hands and face seem puffy and your ankles ache. If you can press into your flesh with a finger and leave a white mark that is a pretty sure sign of it. In fact at least 60–70 per cent of pregnant women have this swelling. It is quite normal. This fluid is a back-up system just in case you should bleed heavily during the birth and it helps to provide an adequate milk flow.

Nevertheless, water retention can increase uncomfortably if you don't get enough rest, and if you blow up suddenly it can be an indication of pre-eclampsia (see page 88). So it should be reported to your doctor or midwife.

You will not be helped by artificially reducing the water retention. 'Water pills' (diuretics), which make you pee more, may be dangerous. You would be better off to take some time off work; take five-minute breaks during the day to put your feet up, or ask a neighbour to look after any other children while you rest.

Stretch marks may appear on your tummy, breasts and thighs. During pregnancy they may look quite dark but they will fade into silvery threads. These marks occur deep down in the lower layers of skin and seem to have more to do with hormones than lack of lubrication. Having someone smooth in cream is extremely unlikely to help but it feels great, relaxes you, and may help to ward off the *itchiness* that some women are plagued with. You don't need expensive creams, anything you like will do.

FEELINGS

'As I grow larger I find that women have started to smile at me in the street. It is as though I am being initiated into a new world – their world. They are saying in those secret smiles, "come on in and join us." I feel closer than ever before to other women. It is our secret, the special part of ourselves which we share, and it crosses all the boundaries of class and race. I feel in love with them all.'

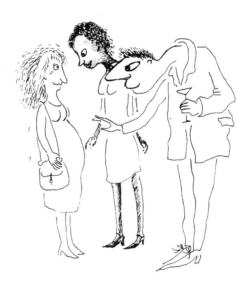

'People talk to my tummy, not to me.'

If you welcome your pregnancy and want to share it you will probably be well rewarded. On the other hand you might find the degree to which you have become public property irritating:

'People talk to my tummy, not to me, they are concerned only about what is happening inside me.'

'I'm really fed up with men who I hardly know feeling that

*they have the right to touch me just because I'm pregnant. At
a meeting the other day this man came charging up to put his
hand on my belly. He would never have dared touch me like
that if I hadn't been pregnant.'*

*'I was at a party recently and a complete stranger came up
and told me that I shouldn't be smoking. I felt like hitting
him. What makes him think that my health is his business?'*

Now that your pregnancy shows you may find yourself being
treated like a piece of glass even though you are probably feeling
better than you have done for weeks.

Changing images and sexuality

Your feelings about your body are an important part of your
sexual identity and the way you present yourself to the world. If
you enjoy the changes that are happening to you, you will find
that others take the same view:

*'Pregnancy was even better than I had expected. I loved
watching my body grow and I was delighted when other
people started to notice and comment about it. Loving my body
spilled over into my sex life. I was happier than I have ever
been.'*

But those changes may not seem so positive:

*'I'd always been so skinny, suddenly developing all these
female characteristics, I couldn't cope with it. I felt depressed,
frightened and rather weird. It wasn't quite my body. There
seemed to be a difference between my body and me.'*

In a society which firmly believes that fat is ugly this can be
quite a difficult time. You may find it hard to feel sexual if you
connect sexuality with being slim and boyish. The images that
surround us shape the way we expect to look and we don't ever
see pictures of naked pregnant women. We certainly don't see
pictures of naked pregnant women making love. In fact you may
well think that it would be disgusting. But pregnancy is the end
result of sex so why are we made to feel that our sexual attrac-
tiveness ends with pregnancy?

If you were very turned off sex in the first three months your confidence may have been shaken. It is quite common for sexual appetite to wane a little during pregnancy. Don't be afraid that your interest in sex has gone for ever. Loving hands rubbing your aching back or smoothing cream on your tummy feels good and comforting, and that is a part of sexual expression.

Fear of sex

Some people are afraid of making love for fear of damaging the baby. If you have been bleeding it is sensible to avoid penetration and orgasm for a couple of weeks, and to avoid the days when you would have had a period in the first few months. If you have had a history of miscarriage you may feel happier avoiding intercourse at least in the first twelve to fourteen weeks (though there isn't any evidence that it makes any difference). If you have painful uterine contractions during orgasm that would also be a reason to avoid it in future.

Apart from these problems, there is no evidence that sex can do anything but good. Orgasm stimulates and exercises the muscles of the uterus; the use of your pelvic floor muscles helps to keep them supple for delivery and afterwards, and loving attention to your nipples will help to prepare them for breastfeeding.

Covering the bulge

Look for clothes which don't dig in and which can be worn without tights or stockings. Even if such a garment would be banned at work, it is worth investing in something soft and stretchy, to sink into when you get home.

Avoid clothes which you may want to wear with high heels as they will put extra strain on your tired back and increase the possibility of damaging it.

You may well be able to save yourself expense by borrowing maternity clothes but try and spare the money for at least one frivolous garment that you feel good in. Something special is happening to your body, so don't hide it, flaunt it.

'IS EVERYTHING ALL RIGHT IN THERE?' PRENATAL SCREENING

At your routine antenatal visits, most of the tests are aimed at ensuring that your health is good and you don't have any conditions which could threaten the health of your baby.

During the middle three months, screening may also be offered to probe inside your womb and see if your baby is handicapped. The evidence collected this way can be very reassuring but it can also be extremely distressing.

Of course the vast majority of women who are screened find that their results are negative. They can continue their pregnancies with an easier mind. But, even for these women, the testing process can be a strain.

Those women who get bad news will then have to decide whether or not to end the pregnancy. Most women opt for abortion in these circumstances but it isn't an easy decision to make, or an easy decision to come to terms with. Penny remembers:

'I thought that I knew what it would mean to have a positive test result but I simply wasn't prepared for it. It's an awful thing to do, to play god, to say this one isn't good enough to live. I had to do it. It wasn't just me, I had my other children to think of too.'

Some women feel that it is better to avoid screening for handicap altogether. They feel that they could cope with caring for a handicapped child if they had one, and they don't want to be faced with the possibility of a distressing choice during pregnancy. This point of view is perfectly valid and should be respected. If you don't want to be screened for 'foetal handicap' during pregnancy you should say so at your first visit to the hospital.

On the other hand, if you do want to be screened, you should make that preference clear also. Only a few hospitals screen automatically and special arrangements may have to be made.

Whichever choice you make, you have a right to full and detailed information, both before the screening process starts, and afterwards. Some hospitals only recall women whose tests are positive but this is a bad practice. You should insist on being contacted personally as soon as the results are known, whether or not they are positive.

If you do get bad news from your test result, don't assume that abortion is the only possibility. Some handicaps are much more disabling than others. The hospital should be able to give you information about this or refer you to someone else who can. Voluntary organisations exist to help the parents of children with almost any disability you can think of. They should be able to give you clear and unbiased advice about what you can expect to face if you decide against abortion.

What are they looking for?

1 **Neural tube defects** (spina bifida, anencephaly, hydrocephaly). These occur in the first weeks of pregnancy when the spinal cord does not form properly. The degree of disability varies. About 50 per cent will be miscarried, half the remainder will be stillborn and many more die in the first year of life. However, of those who survive, 80 per cent will have normal intelligence and of these, 25 per cent will have only a slight physical handicap (about 2 per cent have no obvious handicap at all). The rest will be badly handicapped, usually paralysed below the waist. About 20 per cent will also be brain-damaged.

The chances of carrying a baby with a neural tube defect varies according to where you live, and whether someone in your family, or you yourself, has had one before. It is a bigger problem in Britain than in most other countries, and particularly so in Northern Ireland, the west of Scotland and south Wales. Across the country, between two and three in every 1000 babies are affected. The risk is far greater if you have already had an NTD baby.

2 **Down's syndrome** (mongolism) You are more likely to have a Down's baby as you or your partner get older. The chances increase sharply from about one in 1205 at 25 to one in 365 at the age of 35 and one in 109 at 40. Down's syndrome occurs when the very first process of cell division of the fertilised eggs goes slightly wrong. A Down's baby has noticeably tilted eyes (hence the name mongol), and will be mentally handicapped. About 20 per cent of these babies die at, or soon after, birth because they are prone to heart and intestinal problems.

Amniocentesis (see page 69) will spot most Down's babies. The procedure is carried out at about sixteen weeks of pregnancy. The results take about three weeks.

3 **Other chromosome abnormalities** When the fertilised egg starts to divide, in the first days of pregnancy, mistakes can

occur. These accidents often cause a very early abortion but the embryo may grow without any obvious evidence that anything is wrong. As with Down's syndrome, the chances of abnormal chromosome make-up increases as you get older. These abnormalities are usually picked up during amniocentesis.

4 **Sex-linked hereditary diseases** Diseases such as haemophilia or Duchenne muscular dystrophy are passed on through families to male children only. If you know that your family is affected with a sex-linked hereditary disease, you can discover which sex your baby will be. It might seem terrible to start pregnancy with a 50 per cent chance of a late abortion but a 50 per cent chance may be better than no baby at all. Do make sure you have up to date information about treatments and prospects for babies likely to be born with such a handicap.

The tools and tests

Ultrasound scans are performed routinely in some hospitals three or more times during pregnancy. In other hospitals they are not done at all. Ultrasonic sound waves which cannot be heard by the human ear are beamed into your womb and the pattern of the sound is recorded on video as they bounce off the baby and the placenta. There is no evidence as yet that the procedure is harmful and it is very widely used though it is of course possible that some unforeseen problem may emerge when the process has been in use for a long time.

The video picture is very blurry and needs to be interpreted by a skilled person but it can provide a wide range of very useful information about the following: the length of pregnancy (at twelve weeks a scan can date a pregnancy quite accurately. Later on it is less reliable unless a sequence of scans has been produced throughout pregnancy showing the progress of growth); whether you are carrying more than one baby; the position of the placenta to which the baby is attached; the existence of abnormalities in the shape of your womb, or growths which could obstruct delivery; the sex of the baby (this isn't always possible to determine); visible abnormalities of the growing baby; and as an aid to amniocentesis (see page 69).

At this early stage of pregnancy, you would probably be asked to have plenty to drink before your scan so that your bladder is full. This has the effect of pushing the womb up higher so that it is easier to see. Later in pregnancy an empty bladder may be preferred.

You will be asked to lie flat and your tummy will be greased. Then a machine called a 'transducer' is passed over it. Ask the technician, or doctor, to point out which bit is which if you can't make it out. If you know you are having a scan, see if you can bring your partner with you.

In some hospitals, 'real time' scanning (a continuous picture rather than a single shot) is now so detailed and accurate that it is being used instead of amniocentesis when neural tube defects are suspected. It has the advantage of instant results, no risk of miscarriage, and more detailed information. The technician should be able to give a reasonably accurate assessment of the degree of disability which may help you to decide whether or not to end pregnancy.

In later pregnancy, the scan can also spot potential problems such as *placenta praevia* (see page 88), allowing time for a Cae-sarean delivery before the baby's life is threatened. Some women might find this information a reassuring back-up if they are keen to have an uncomplicated home, or GP unit delivery.

An alpha-feto-protein test is carried out at seventeen weeks. It is a blood test to discover how much AFP is given off your baby into your bloodstream. As your pregnancy progresses, so the AFP level in your blood increases. At seventeen weeks it is possible to see whether the AFP level is higher than it should be.

A raised AFP level could mean that your pregnancy is fur-ther on than you realised (it is important to be accurate about your dates if this test is to mean anything), or that you are carrying more than one baby (an ultrasound scan will check that). However in some cases it may indicate the presence of a baby with a neural tube defect (see page 66). If your AFP is raised you would be referred for more tests to see if the baby is affected.

In some areas, these blood tests are given routinely to every-one. In others they are not offered at all unless you have a family history of NTD. Even when they are not offered, you may be able to get the test if you ask at the right time. Where the tests are routine, you should have an equal right to refuse it if you would rather not know.

If your AFP is high, you should be given a second test, just to be sure, followed by an ultrasound scan. If a real time scanner is used the technician will be able to tell immediately whether or not your baby has a neural tube defect. In other hospitals, older equipment can only tell whether or not you are having twins, and double check your dates.

If the ultrasound scan was not sensitive enough to pick up NTDs, you will now have an amniocentesis. Only about one in every ten women who have amniocentesis for a raised AFP will be told that the test does indeed show evidence of a neural tube defect. There is a tiny possibility of a false positive with amniocentesis but with recent, more sophisticated, screening techniques the chances of that are only one in every 200,000 women screened. However, as you will see below, amniocentesis carries other risks, so ultrasound scanning is clearly preferable if good enough equipment and trained staff are available.

Even if you have been through all this, there is still a slight chance that your baby will be born with a neural tube defect. The screening system does miss a few NTD babies.

Amniocentesis is a test of the amniotic fluid in which the baby is floating. The test cannot be carried out earlier than the sixteenth week of pregnancy because there will not be enough liquid to allow for it to be safely drawn off. If you leave it much later than this, and add on the three weeks necessary to test the sample for chromosome defects (longer if the culture has to be done again which can happen), it is getting a bit late for an abortion should you feel it is necessary.

Amniocentesis is done by putting a long hollow needle into the womb and drawing amniotic fluid through it. The place where the needle will be inserted is first numbed with a local anaesthetic. The procedure is not painful though some women find it disturbing and unpleasant. Penny remembers,

'I felt naked and worried about the baby. I felt I was putting us both at risk. I wanted them just to go away and stop doing it. The three-week wait for results was terrible. I became more anxious every day.'

Risks of amniocentesis   The procedure should only be carried out when an ultrasound scan can also be used to show the exact position of the baby or the placenta and ensure that the needle does not touch the placenta.

Large studies of the procedure show an increased risk of

miscarriage after amniocentesis. Between one and four babies in every 200 miscarry, and there is a similar increase in the number of babies being born with unexplained breathing difficulties and limb abnormalities. With ultrasound, the risk of miscarriage is reduced.

Given these drawbacks, it is clearly not sensible to offer amniocentesis routinely to all women. It is up to each person, with help and advice from medical staff, to make their own decision.

Weighing it up For reasons which have not yet been discovered, even apparently normal babies who give out high levels of AFP are more vulnerable than most, so the chances of a miscarriage during amniocentesis is somewhat higher than normal. Nevertheless, with a one in ten chance of bearing a baby with a neural tube defect, your need to know for certain will probably outweigh your concern about the procedure. You could ask whether a 'real time scan' could be done instead of amniocentesis though the necessary technology may not yet be available locally.

If you want to check on Down's syndrome or any of the other chromosome disorders the risks and benefits are harder to weigh up (see page 66). If you are over 38, the chances of having a Down's baby are higher than the chances of miscarrying a normal one. In America, all women over 35 are offered the chance of screening; in Britain the age for routine screening varies between 35 and 39. If you are, say, 37, and feel that amniocentesis would make the difference between a happy confident pregnancy and a miserable scared one, then it is probably worth it in emotional terms. If you would simply rather not think about it, don't. Marie was single and 35 when she was offered amniocentesis. The result was negative.

'Before my pregnancy I'd always intended to have all the tests done. When I was told about the risks of miscarriage it really shook me. It seemed crazy to go through a procedure which carried four times as high a risk of miscarriage as of finding an abnormality. But then when I thought about the consequences of having a mongol child, and probably having to give it to the state to care for, I decided to go ahead with it and I am very glad I did.'

Fetoscopy and trophoblast sampling are two new procedures which are only in their experimental stages. At present both of them carry a high risk for the developing baby and they are unlikely to be offered.

Ending a pregnancy

A late induced abortion is a pretty harrowing experience whatever the reason for it. A substance called prostaglandin will be injected into your womb, or fed by a tube, through your cervix. Prostaglandin makes your womb contract as it does in labour to push the baby out.

The contractions are painful and may go on for up to twelve hours, or possibly more. You should discuss the question of pain relief with the doctor who should ensure that the experience is made as easy for you as possible.

Afterwards you will need a great deal of loving support. Don't bottle your feelings up, find someone to talk to and don't hide your unhappiness from your partner either. You will both need the opportunity to grieve.

Penny had already had three children when, during her fourth pregnancy, she was told that her baby would have Down's syndrome. An abortion was arranged for her the next day so there was no time for second thoughts.

'When I arrived at the hospital for the abortion, no one seemed to know why I was there, I had to tell them. The doctor had said that I wouldn't know much about it but, after the first couple of hours when I was given something to knock me out, I was fully conscious and all alone. It wasn't bad pain, but I cried a lot, and the nurses were horrid.

I wouldn't look at the baby when it came. I wish I had done now. I don't think I would be so haunted by it if I'd really known what it looked like. Next morning, when it was all over, everyone was very kind. I felt quite elated, just as I do after a normal birth, but three days later the milk came and I went to pieces.

For six months I was very depressed. I would wake at night and go downstairs to cry. Finally, I went to a very sympathetic woman doctor who put me on anti-depressants, and I was able to make some decisions about my life. I knew that I had to have another baby. This time I told nobody, not even the other children, that I was pregnant. I had decided to have amniocentesis again. It was almost as though I needed to confirm my earlier decision. To prove to myself that I had done the right thing.'

Penny's next baby was quite healthy and is much loved. Looking back, she feels that she made the right decision, but it was a very hard one to make.

MATERNITY RIGHTS: USING THE LAW

'I'd been there three years so I was entitled to maternity leave but I didn't have it easy. I had quite a few days off sick and then I had to go into hospital because I was bleeding, something to do with the placenta, I was six months then and I was going back until I was seven and a half months but they said "Don't come back" more or less. Whilst I was in hospital they had fixed up someone else to do my job anyway. There were a lot of arguments and hassles. In the end they did pay it but there was a lot of aggro.'

(From *Pregnant at Work* by Sue Rodwell and Liz Smart, Open University, 1982)

Maternity rights at work

Compared to other countries in Europe we get very little help from the state when we have babies. In Sweden, for example, both parents of a new baby have a right to share a paid leave entitlement of nine months plus an extra three months unpaid. They also have the right to reduce their working hours while their children are below school age.

In Britain what little we get in the way of cash and job security is wound up in a mass of red tape. It is vital to find out exactly what you are entitled to or you may lose your right to return to work. Below are set out on one side the rights which exist in law, on the other the people who are entitled to them. If you are at all concerned about your own position, you should read a more detailed guide (see page 201) or get help from your union, a legal advice centre, or a citizen's advice bureau.

Some employers have demonstrated that they will not hesitate to deprive women of their jobs if they fail to comply with the notification procedures to the letter. If you wish to protect your rights to return to work you must notify your employer that you want to return. If you are not certain how you will feel once the baby is born then leave your options open by saying that you want your job back.

Your right to job protection and cash

The rights

Maternity grant of £25 can be claimed on form BM4. Send also an 'Expected date of confinement' form signed by your midwife or doctor.

Both forms are available from a clinic or local social security office.

Maternity allowance is a weekly benefit paid for up to eighteen weeks. It is the same amount as unemployment benefit (£25 in 1983). Claim on the same forms and at the same time as for maternity grant (above). If you are single you may be able to claim for extra dependants so check with your social security office.

The benefit is paid for eleven weeks before the birth and seven weeks after. If you stay on later at work, or the baby comes early, you lose the benefit for the missed weeks. If the baby is late, you get more. (If you are forced to leave earlier you can claim for sickness benefit.)

You must apply between week 26 and week 29 to avoid losing benefit.

Who gets them

Any woman who is more than twenty-eight weeks pregnant.

You qualify for this money if you have paid full national insurance contributions in the year *before* you became pregnant. The contributions year runs from April to April so look back to the April before you became pregnant, it is the year up to that which counts. You will need also, on 1982 figures, to have paid contributions on income of at least £1350. It is complicated; if you aren't sure, apply anyway and let them sort it out.

Maternity pay is 90 per cent of your basic rate of pay, minus the maternity allowance (above) which will be deducted whether you claim for it or not. The money is refunded to your employer by the government. It is a right, not a favour, and you are entitled to it whether or not you intend to return to work.

If you qualify for maternity pay you must inform your employer, in writing, at least twenty-one days before you intend to leave work (or as soon as you can if ill health forces you to leave earlier). You may also be requested to provide an 'expected date of confinement' form signed by a doctor or midwife.

The money can be paid weekly or in a lump sum and you are entitled to all of it even if you work later than eleven weeks before the birth.

You are eligible for maternity pay if you have been employed continuously with your current employer for two years up to the eleventh week before your baby is due. If you work between eight and sixteen hours a week you will need to have worked for five continuous years (on fewer hours you don't qualify).

You may not leave work earlier than the eleventh week before the baby is due unless (a) you are on holiday, (b) you are off sick (with a sick note), or (c) you have been legally dismissed (see page 47), but would have qualified if you hadn't been.

Previous maternity leaves with the same employer count as part of continuous employment.

Getting your job back
You have the right to return to work up to twenty-nine weeks after your baby is born. (Count the week of the birth as week one.) You are then entitled to be employed on terms and conditions which are as good as those you left (including any pay rises which would have been due).

If your employer finds it impractical to give you your

You qualify for job security on the same grounds as for maternity pay (above). However there are other restrictions.

1 If your employer has five or fewer employees he can refuse to take you back if he finds it 'impractical' to keep your job open. He would have to prove that it was impractical so it is still worth

own job back you must be offered a suitable alternative. It is very important to check now that the job description in your contract of employment actually describes the job you do. That should restrict 'suitable alternatives' to similar jobs.

If you refuse the alternative job you will lose your right to any job.

If your job disappears due to redundancy, you are entitled to an alternative or, failing that, to redundancy pay. Again, you cannot refuse the alternative job.

Your employer can delay your return to work by a month. If you are not well enough to return to work after twenty-nine weeks, you can, on production of a medical certificate, put off your return for a month.

If there is a strike or lay-off at the time you expected to return to work, you must still write the letters and start as soon as it's over.

a try.

2 When you apply for maternity pay (see above), you must inform your employer, in writing, twenty-one days before you intend to stop work, that you are having the baby and intend to return to work. You must also give the expected date of confinement and you may be asked to supply a signed form from your doctor or midwife.

3 If your employer writes to you, not sooner than seven weeks after the expected date of the birth, asking you to write and confirm your intention to return to work, YOU MUST REPLY WITHIN FOURTEEN DAYS, or you could forfeit your rights to return.

4 You must write to your employer at least twenty-one days before you intend to return to work giving the date you will come back.

If you don't qualify

If you have no legal right to your job back your employer may be prepared to make a special exception:

'I didn't know much but they said because I supervised the other girls, that they'd hold my job open. We don't work

enough hours for our jobs to be left open really. I went to see the manager and he said by the time it'd take for him to train someone else it'd be easier to wait for me to come back.' (from Pregnant at Work)

In some cases your trade union may already have negotiated maternity rights which do not have a long qualifying period, according to *Bargaining Report 8* (published by the Labour Research Department). In thirty-six out of fifty agreements studied companies gave paid maternity leave after one year's service. These included the Post Office, the BBC, local authorities, British Airways, Butlins and Rowntree Mackintosh. In some companies, part-timers are entitled to paid leave. Unpaid leave of a year or more may also be available.

It is probably too late for you to get your negotiated agreement changed now but your experience may encourage your union to fight harder for improved maternity rights the next time round.

Paternity leave

'Paternity leave? No I don't think we should provide that, most men want to get as far away as possible when there is a new baby in the house' (a comment from management in a big publishing company).

In spite of attitudes like these, surveys show that the majority of fathers do take some time off around the time of a birth. More and more trade unions are now including some period of paternity leave in their negotiations and the more progressive employers have recognised that their male employees do need some consideration at such an important moment of their lives. Nevertheless, a recent survey compiled for the Equal Opportunities Commission showed that the vast majority of men had to use paid leave entitlement in order to be around when their babies were born.

Even the employers and trade unions who do recognise that men want to be in at the birth usually see it as a way of helping the mother. In fact, if women are to have true equality at work, it stands to reason that they should not be expected to take on the full burden of child care at home. However, the Swedish concept of equal entitlements so that men can share in the up-bringing of their children, is still very far from the minds of law makers, employers and, to a large extent, trade unionists as well.

A flexible return to work

'I have to go back to work but I just cannot face leaving Alice every day, all day, I wish I could reduce my hours but I think I've left it too late. I just hope the others will understand if I slip away early.'

Babies get to you. Jill had taken advantage of a generous maternity leave during which she was rarely parted from her new baby for more than a couple of hours. The thought of going back to work full-time was causing her enormous anxiety and ruining the last few weeks of her leave. Her experience is extremely common. Too few women have been through the experience of taking maternity leave for the wisdom to be passed on properly. Each new batch find the same problems staring them in the face when they have to face the wrench of separation.

One of the most useful things you could do now is raise with your employer the possibility of a phased return to work. You have no legal right to return on anything other than the conditions on which you left but you may be able to exchange a month working part time for an earlier return to work. You will probably find that it is well worth it.

Job sharing could be a good option. Contact the Job Sharing Project (see page 204) for information on the practical and contractual problems involved.

CLASSES

'For this birth I attended NCT classes. This time I practised my breathing and learned about how my body works during labour. The pelvic floor exercises were particularly helpful. I did them twice each day for the last month and I am sure that is why I recovered so quickly down there. With this baby I didn't have the 'everything is falling out' feeling that I got toward the end of my last pregnancy and after the birth. Nor did I suffer from piles this time.'

Childbirth (or parentcraft classes) will be held at your hospital or clinic. You may prefer to attend National Childbirth Trust classes (see page 204 for address) which charge a small fee (they will sometimes drop the fee if you are very short of money).

At the hospital you will be told about the system which will be used, you will see the labour and delivery room, meet the staff who will care for you, and have the opportunity to ask questions about their methods.

At NCT classes (which are held in private houses) and clinics, you will meet women from the immediate area who are going through it all with you. The NCT groups organise reunions and postnatal support groups which can provide you with a ready-made circle of friends. That can be a life saver if you are alone at home for the first time.

A good class will include your partner or chosen companion. It will encourage you to approach childbirth without fear; teach you methods of relaxation and ways of coping with labour with the minimum amount of drugs; discuss methods of pain relief so that you have full information when the time comes to decide whether you need help; and describe the stages of labour and the physical changes in your body and, finally breastfeeding and baby care.

If your hospital class spends four lessons discussing birth technology and drugs and only one on breathing techniques, the stages of labour and breastfeeding, you may be better off with the NCT. Of course you can always go to both.

Learning together with your partner or birth companion can make a big difference to the experience of labour for both of you. Attending a birth with somebody you care for may be distressing if you don't know what is going on. A companion who understands how best to help will not only feel more able to participate, he or she will also be able to protect you against unwanted attention and help you to decide when you do need help.

If your partner, or companion, cannot get to classes it will help to read the chapter on birth in this book.

Sharing your fears could make them smaller. You will find that most other women are nervous about labour. The group atmosphere of the NCT classes may also make it easier to say things that you find hard to discuss with your partner.

'I always felt that he thought I was making a fuss. Once he

heard other women saying how tired they felt, and how much they needed help, he was more attentive. I started to feel that I had a right to ask to be cared for.'

A woman alone may feel at a disadvantage in an NCT class. Said Fiona, 'I know it was irrational, but I hated the cosiness of it, it felt like an advertisement for compulsory heterosexuality.' Nevertheless, she was glad she had been. 'Those classes were a great comfort through a twenty-four hour labour.'

Techniques for coping with labour vary with each teacher. We have explained one system in the chapter on birth. If you cannot get to classes the explanation will probably help.

Chapter 4

THE STRANDED WHALE

28–40 weeks

'I didn't dare buy any clothes for the baby until now. I couldn't really believe that the pregnancy would work. Now that I've been pregnant for twenty-eight weeks, I know that I am going to have a baby.'

How does it grow?

28 weeks   Other people can now feel the baby moving inside you as its feet and hands knock against the walls of the womb. Your baby would stand a good chance of surviving if it was born tomorrow, provided it was delivered in a hospital with good intensive care facilities, but it would be tiny. It still needs to gain twice its current weight before it is completely ready for birth and it would have difficulty breathing without help.

32 weeks   By now the movements are clearly visible to others. You can probably pick out which end is the head and which is the bottom and locate feet and hands as they punch the walls of your womb.

In the next fortnight or so your baby will probably turn round, head down, and stay that way for the rest of your pregnancy. If it doesn't do so, you can encourage it by spending ten minutes, twice a day, lying on your back with your legs over your ears, or raising your hips up on cushions.

36 weeks   If this is your first baby, during the next four weeks the head will move right down into your pelvis (*engage*) ready for the birth. If you have already had one child, this one will probably not engage until labour starts. If you, or your parents, come from Africa you may find that your first baby doesn't engage until labour starts either. This is usually perfectly normal and happens because your pelvic bones are a slightly different shape. (If your first baby's head does not come down, check the paragraph on pelvic disproportion, page 92.)

You may notice an odd feeling rather like a ticking clock just above your pubic bone. That is just the baby having an attack of hiccups!

Pregnancy officially lasts forty weeks from the first day of your last period. The baby will then be about thirty-eight weeks old. The majority of births take place within two weeks before, or after, that time.

How does it lie?

Towards the end of your pregnancy the position, or lie, of the baby will be noted at every antenatal check. A baby which is unusually placed will have a more difficult time getting out and you may have to discuss with midwives and doctors at the hospital just how the delivery should best be handled.

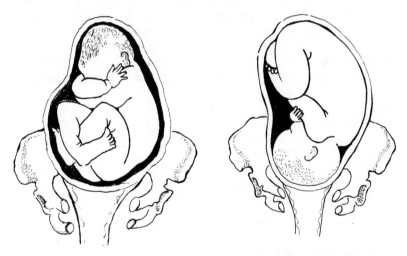

Breech presentation   *Cephalic (vertex) presentation*

Here is an explanation of the notes which the midwife will probably make on your card to indicate the lie, presentation (see below) and position of your baby. The short form which will probably be noted on your card is in brackets.

The lie
Longitudinal (L) means that the baby is lying head up or down. *Transverse* (Trans) *or Oblique* (unstable lie) means that it is lying across your tummy (see page 92.)

The presentation
Cephalic (Ceph) means the head is pointing down. Usually the baby's head is well tucked in and the right way round. This is referred to as Vertex (Vx).

Breech (Br) means its bottom is pointing down (see page 90).

The position
The way that the baby faces is also noted. Labour is easiest if the baby is facing towards your backbone. This position is described either as a left, or a right, *occipito anterior* (L/ROA). If the baby is facing towards your tummy, or sideways, it will be described as *posterior*, or *lateral* (L/ROP or L/ROL).

Most babies turn into the anterior position before labour starts. If a 'posterior' baby doesn't turn round, it will usually try to do so during labour. This can cause what is known as a 'backache' labour which may be longer and tends to stop and start. Knowing which way your baby is facing could make a difference to your choice of method of pain relief, if any (see page 128).

Movements

Once the baby's head has engaged, there is less space to move in, so you may notice that the baby is less active. You are right to take note of movements, particularly towards the end of pregnancy, as these are important indicators of your baby's health (see page 95).

HOW DO YOU FEEL?

'Sometimes I feel I need a winch to help me turn over at night. Getting in and out of bed to go to the toilet several times a night is quite an effort. The mattress springs have given out under the strain.'

Most of the discomforts of these last few weeks have already been described in the last section (pages 54–62). You may feel new ones too.

Amnesia   *'I went into the greengrocer's for a pound of Cox's. When I opened my mouth nothing came out. I had forgotten the word.'* Susan was experiencing 'maternal amnesia', when you keep forgetting things and get confused. Some women find that their memory comes back after the birth. Others feel that it is never quite the same again.

Braxton Hicks contractions are practice contractions which you will probably feel as tightening sensations across your belly. They are getting the womb ready for labour and happen all through pregnancy but become more frequent, and much more noticeable, as you get nearer to the birth.

Breathlessness can be a problem because your uterus is pressing against your diaphragm and compressing your lungs.

Indigestion and heartburn are common in late pregnancy (see page 56).

Frequent peeing may wake you several times a night in the last few weeks as your baby's head moves down into your pelvis squashing your bladder. You will probably notice that this change is accompanied by an improvement in your heartburn and breathlessness.

Occasionally you may feel an urge to pee which goes away as soon as you get to a toilet. This may be a Braxton Hicks contraction forcing the baby's head down on your bladder. Next time, put your hand on your tummy, and see if the urge to pee is accompanied by a tightening feeling. If it is, just wait for it to pass, and the feeling will die away.

Swollen and aching ankles are a common worry. They swell because the bump of your tummy is slowing down the rate at which liquid is pumped back up your legs. Try sitting with your feet up to allow gravity to help. See Water retention, page 61.

Tingling fingers are caused by fluid retention pressing down on the nerves in your wrist. This is called carpal tunnel syndrome. Try raising the arm above your head for a few minutes to ease it. It may be a sign that you need more rest.

Shooting pains down your thighs or in your pelvis are caused by your baby's head pinching a nerve against your pubic bone.

Constipation may get worse towards the end of pregnancy as your bowel is compressed (see page 57).

Piles may also get worse now. Turn back to page 57 for suggestions.

Backache may be caused by the extra weight at the front. It helps to get down on all fours and take the weight off your spine.

Sleeplessness may be due to discomfort or plain worry. Some women find themselves lying awake for no particular reason. Try to avoid sleeping pills which will go through to the baby. Get up and make yourself a warm milk drink. It will make you drowsy as well as boosting your calcium supply. Camomile tea is another gentle sleep inducer. You can buy it in health food shops and some chemists. You may find that a walk in the late afternoon will help you to sleep. The worst thing you can do about sleeplessness is to worry about it. Tessa recalls,

'I expected to be a little wakeful towards the end of pregnancy. I would just keep a book by the bed and read for a while. It never worried me.'

Preparing your body for the birth

Rest is not a waste of time. You need it. You have a right to leave work at twenty-eight weeks. If you have the energy to work beyond that time you can do so but don't be too hard on yourself. If you find your face and ankles swelling with fluid retention it is usually a sign to take things a bit easier. If your blood pressure is up you should definitely stop work.

If you are at home with a toddler to care for, you could try to arrange a swop with a friend, which will give you a short break during the day. You may be tempted to use the time to clean the kitchen. Try to resist it. Leave the housework to someone else or, if there is no one else to do it, keep it to the minimum. (How about a supply of paper plates for the days when you are extra tired?)

Food in these last weeks is particularly important. Your baby's weight will triple in the last three months. It is also an important time for brain development. Even if you feel that you have put on too much weight, don't stop eating now, you can work on losing the weight once the baby is born. Look back to the section on food in Chapter 1 (page 1). If you don't have the energy for cooking, or a partner to do it, stock up with good things that don't take too much attention. Muesli, porridge, wholemeal bread, cheeses, large potatoes for baking, vegetables that need little preparation, fruit, nuts, yoghurt, eggs and milk.

'I lived on baked potatoes with cheese in them for most of my pregnancy,' says Micky. If you get bored with that, try Lynn's recipe: 'Whisk an egg, a banana and a spoon of wheatgerm (available from many chemists) into a pint of milk. Hey presto – a nourishing, easily digested meal that doesn't even dirty any dishes.'

Practise squatting for a few minutes each day to strengthen your thigh muscles just in case you want to give birth in this position. Squatting also helps to stretch the *perineum*, the skin between your anus and vagina, which needs to stretch, without tearing, during delivery.

Massaging oil into your *perineum* (see above) may also help to make it more elastic.

Relaxation is something you (and your partner) can learn to do now. It will help you during labour and will be invaluable after the baby is born. If you go to birth preparation classes, you will be shown how to relax.

1 Sit in a straight backed chair with your hands in your lap. Close your eyes and concentrate very hard on your hands, willing them to get warmer. You will find that they actually do warm up, but more important, the concentration will blank everything else from your mind, slow your breathing, and help you to feel relaxed. It is a very good technique to use while waiting in antenatal clinics!

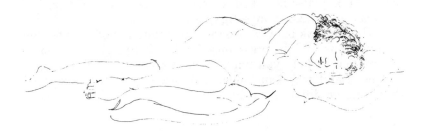

2 Lie down on your side with your top leg forward supported on a cushion (see illustration). Now take a deep slow breath and stretch your leg down towards your heel (don't point your toes) so that the muscles tense all the way up. Then blow out slowly

and gradually relax. Take another deep breath and move on right up through your body, breathing in, and out, and tensing and then relaxing all your muscles separately, paying special attention to your shoulders and face. After this you may well find yourself dropping off to sleep.

Travelling is best kept to a minimum in late pregnancy. Long journeys can be very tiring. If you need to travel, take frequent breaks to stretch your legs and stimulate your blood circulation. Airlines will not let you fly after thirty-six weeks.

KNOWING WHEN YOU NEED HELP

For most women, pregnancy and childbirth are perfectly normal events, which proceed from beginning to end without the need for anything other than routine antenatal checks and an experienced midwife to assist during the birth.

For some 4500 women in this country each year, pregnancy is medically managed, and one month or more is spent in hospital under the close scrutiny of doctors.

In between these two groups lie a large number of women who experience some difficulty in pregnancy and need to make decisions about whether they require, and are willing to accept, the various treatments which are available.

The most likely decisions you might be called upon to make are: whether to go into hospital; whether to accept an induction (artificially triggered labour); whether to have a Caesarean section. You may also be asked to agree to take certain drugs; and to ultrasound or X-ray investigation.

What follows is by no means a complete list of the possible complications of late pregnancy but it should give you some information to help you make decisions for yourself. Where it will be useful we've included, in brackets, the usual medical shorthand for different conditions.

High blood pressure (↑ BP or H/T)

In the last three months your blood pressure will be checked regularly – every fortnight, at first, and then weekly. In about 10 per cent of first pregnancies and 5 per cent of subsequent pregnancies, blood pressure rises above the level considered normal for you (see page 44).

Your blood pressure may rise in pregnancy because you already have a tendency to high blood pressure. Pregnancy may trigger it off or make it worse. The rise may be due to a specific condition of pregnancy known as pre-eclampsia or pre-eclamptic toxaemia (PET). Or it may be a temporary change due to passing anxiety.

Although you will probably be quite unaware of these conditions in their earlier stages, both high blood pressure and pre-eclampsia can be dangerous to both mother and baby and this is why they are so carefully monitored.

How does it affect the baby? While your blood pressure is high you are not pumping blood into the placenta at the best possible rate. This means that the baby is getting less than the maximum amount of food from you. If the high blood pressure is severe, and lasts, it may also restrict the oxygen supply to the baby. This means that you have a greater chance of having a baby who is small and could become distressed during labour. This problem could be worse if you also smoke.

This does not mean that your baby will necessarily be in danger. If the blood pressure is only a little bit higher than normal, the risks are only marginally higher than they would be for a woman with normal blood pressure. Even women with very high blood pressure are more likely than not to produce healthy babies, but the risk of problems is twice what it would be for women with normal blood pressure.

If the rise in your blood pressure is not stopped and you reach the stage of eclamptic fits, both you and your baby would be in grave danger. Fortunately this stage is very rarely reached if the problem is recognised early and that is what antenatal care is for. The symptoms of impending eclampsia are: severe headaches; flashing lights; nausea, vomiting or pain in the abdomen. If you experience any of them, contact your doctor or midwife for an immediate blood pressure check. If eclampsia is suspected, your baby will need to be delivered quickly.

Temporary raised blood pressure may simply be caused by anxiety, as Cathy discovered:

'The last six weeks of pregnancy were miserable. Every time I went to the clinic my blood pressure was up. When my midwife checked it at home it was fine. I was fortunate to have

a midwife who agreed to care for me at home. I'm sure that if they had taken me into hospital as they wanted to my blood pressure would have stayed up permanently.'

Doctors say that the lower (diastolic) number of your blood pressure will not be affected by momentary stress but the experience of women in pregnancy seems to throw doubt on this. If your blood pressure does go up at one visit (particularly if you had a long and stressful wait) try the 'hands in the lap' relaxation mentioned on page 85 while you are waiting for the next check. If the rise was just caused by anxiety you may be able to keep it down this way.

Pre-eclampsia is suspected if the lower number of your blood pressure rises above 90 for two consecutive checks (unless you had high blood pressure at the start of pregnancy), particularly if this is accompanied by protein in your urine (see page 39) and/or water retention (oedema, see page 61).

If the lower number rises above 100, or there is protein in your urine, you may be advised to go into hospital for rest and observation. (Some doctors disagree; see below). If the figure goes over 110 coupled with protein in your urine the baby may need to be delivered, as it will probably do better in a special care unit than inside you.

The treatment of pre-eclampsia

There are many different theories about the causes of pre-eclampsia and its treatment. In the early stages you can do a great deal to help yourself. From the information available the following seems to be the safest way of caring for yourself and your baby:

1 **A good diet** Some women restrict their diets to try and avoid excess weight gain in late pregnancy. There is evidence to suggest that this restriction does more harm than good. If your blood pressure rises, make certain that you are eating a good range of protein, fresh fruit and vegetables and some starch foods. If you cut back drastically on starch your body will have to use up protein supplies to make energy. In late pregnancy you need extra energy, as well as extra protein.

2 **Salt** In the past, doctors wrongly believed that cutting your salt intake could cut down on the water retention which accompanied pre-eclampsia. Indeed a British study way back in 1958 showed that women who ate salt freely were less likely to get

pre-eclampsia and that some women who developed early symptoms were relieved of them by increasing their salt intake.

3 **Rest** is always advised if any of the symptoms of pre-eclampsia occur. According to an article in *The British Medical Journal* in 1978, there is no need for complete bed rest or hospital admission, unless the lower (diastolic) blood pressure climbs as high as 110 with protein in the urine too. Rest at home is usually more relaxing and it is relaxation that you need.

You may feel full of energy but your body is telling you to slow down. If you can't sleep during the day, use the relaxation exercises mentioned on page 85. When you are resting, lie on your side, rather than your back, to keep the weight off the large blood vessels which feed your placenta.

If you have not yet stopped working outside your home you would be wise to do so now, and if you have other children, speak to your health visitor who may be able to arrange for them to be cared for while you get a break each day.

4 **Diuretics** (water pills) are sometimes suggested but studies suggest that they are positively harmful.

The anxiety double bind If you are a worrier, and perhaps nervous about the birth itself, adding the problem of high blood pressure will probably make you feel even more anxious. One of the best ways of dealing with anxiety is finding someone to talk to about it. If medical staff seem too busy to spend time with you, contact the National Childbirth Trust teacher in your area, or the Pre-eclamptic Toxaemia Society. They may well be able to find someone locally who has time to chat and calm your anxieties (see page 204 for addresses).

Bleeding in late pregnancy

Contact your doctor or midwife if you start to bleed and, if the bleeding is heavy, or accompanied by pain, you should ring the hospital direct and ask for the emergency obstetric unit.

Slight bleeding, uncomplicated by pain, may be caused by one of the minor problems on page 22. However it could be much more serious than that so don't just ignore it and hope it will go away.

After twenty-eight weeks any bleeding from the womb is called an ante-partum haemorrhage. There are two major causes of bleeding: 1 **Abruptio placenta**, when the placenta, to which the baby is attached, comes away from the wall of the womb. This puts both mother and baby at risk and would need urgent medical attention. This condition is usually accompanied by pain. 2 **Placenta praevia** when the placenta is covering the neck of the womb, causing bleeding which is usually painless and may stop and start.

Treatment for bleeding
Your midwife or doctor will visit and arrange for you to be admitted into hospital to discover the cause of the bleeding and its possible effect on the baby. If you have lost a lot of blood you will be given a blood transfusion.

Now an ultrasound scan will check the position of the placenta. If it is overlapping the neck of your womb, arrangements will probably be made for a Caesarean section, at about thirty-eight weeks. You may be kept in hospital until the delivery to ensure that you don't go into labour and tear the placenta which would endanger you both.

If the placenta doesn't completely cover the neck of the womb you would be examined, under anaesthetic, to see whether a normal delivery would be possible. If it isn't, a Caesarean may be performed while you are still under the anaesthetic so you should discuss this possibility with the doctor (see page 101).

If the placenta is coming away the treatment will depend on the amount of separation. If it is slight, and the baby is still kicking vigorously, with a good heartbeat, you will simply be kept in hospital. Regular checks will be made on the baby's health. If there is any sign that the placenta is failing, early delivery will be suggested (see page 97).

If the bleeding is severe, or you are clearly very ill, the baby would be delivered as soon as possible by Caesarean.

Breech presentation (B)

If your baby is one of the three babies in every hundred which end up feet, or bottom down, you will have to discuss the management of your labour very carefully with your consultant. You will definitely need to give birth in hospital. There is a risk, for example, that the cord may be squashed while the baby's head is being delivered. If delivery is delayed, this could block the baby's oxygen supply, so emergency back-up is essential.

Turning it round, external cephalic version, as it is called, may be tried (unless you have high blood pressure, which increases the chance of haemorrhage). This requires skill to ensure that the placenta is not damaged. You will be asked to lie on a couch, possibly with a raised end, to encourage the baby to 'float' up as high as possible out of the ring of your pelvic bones. Then the doctor will place one hand on the baby's head and the other on its bottom while turning it gently. Some babies turn straight back again afterwards.

You could try encouraging it to turn yourself. Do not, under any circumstances, attempt to push, or manipulate it. You could tear the placenta and endanger both your own and the baby's life. Lie with your abdomen propped up on pillows for ten minutes twice a day and gently stroke and talk your baby into moving. If the baby does turn, squat down, or walk around to give it a chance to settle down firmly.

Delivery In Britain a cut is usually made (episiotomy) and forceps used to protect the head and speed delivery. An early induction may also be suggested to ensure that the baby's head is still quite flexible and will 'mould' easily on the way out. One clinic at Pithiviers, in France, delivers breech babies without episiotomies, or any other intervention, while the mother is standing. However this is unlikely to happen in the UK.

A *Caesarean* is possible, particularly if this is your first baby. About 40 per cent of breech babies are delivered in this way.

Studies show that breech babies do about equally well delivered either way. The safest delivery for you is probably the one that your consultant feels safest doing.

Twins

Twins occur in one out of every ninety pregnancies. Identical twins, when a single egg splits at the first stage of development, are random happenings but you are more likely to have non-identical twins if there are already some in your family on your mother's side.

If you are carrying more than one baby, your body will be under greater strain. You are more likely to suffer from minor discomforts and from pregnancy complications. Your babies are also more likely to be premature. You should take great care of yourself. Eat as well as you can, and take plenty of rest. If your work involves heavy lifting or a lot of standing you would do well to seek a transfer. Discuss your work with your doctor or midwife and ask for advice on this.

You may be asked to go into hospital between 28 and 32 weeks because of an increased risk of going into labour. Once past this stage, the risk subsides and you can go home again. If you feel you would get more rest at home, ask if you can stay at home and be visited by a district midwife.

Delivery of twins need not be much more complicated than a single birth but it should take place in hospital because there is an increased risk for the second baby if it isn't born swiftly. You may be encouraged to accept an epidural anaesthetic (see page 131) in case forceps are required for the second twin. If one of them is lying in the breech position forceps will almost certainly be used. However, if they are both head down, this may not be necessary and you could opt to manage without drugs.

Unstable lie

If your baby keeps changing position in the last weeks of pregnancy you will probably be asked to go into hospital early to ensure that you don't go into labour with the baby wedged in an awkward position. The contractions may push the baby into position during the first stage of labour if it's badly placed. If labour starts with the baby lying across your tummy you will probably need a Caesarean.

Small pelvis/big baby (cephalo pelvic disproportion, or CPD)

If the circle of your pelvic bones seems too narrow to allow a baby to pass through, a Caesarean section will be recommended.

In the last couple of weeks of pregnancy, the midwife or doctor will check to see whether the baby's head has engaged. To do this they note the amount of the head that can be felt above the pubic bone. If the head is fully engaged (eng.) you should be all right, if there is any doubt about the size of your pelvis, in relation to your baby's head, an X-ray may be suggested. In general X-rays should be avoided in pregnancy, but at this late stage it is unlikely to harm the baby, and may save you from having an unnecessary Caesarean.

An early induction may also be suggested so that the baby would be born while its head was still flexible enough to squeeze through, or you may be allowed to wait for labour to start naturally, provided you don't go beyond your due date. The 'trial of labour', as it is called, would be carefully monitored and, if it did not progress satisfactorily, you would be delivered by Caesarean.

Premature labour

If you feel pain at any time during pregnancy you should report it. It may be nothing more than indigestion. If it is early labour, you will probably have a pretty strong suspicion yourself. Listen to your body. You are your own best monitor. (See page 111.)

If this is premature labour you need to get yourself into hospital as quickly as possible so that, if the baby is delivered, it will get the best possible care.

Go to the hospital where you are booked. You may be transferred from there to a bigger hospital with intensive care facilities. If you are not at home when the contractions start, head for the nearest maternity hospital. You should have your Coop card with you at all times for just such an eventuality.

Treatment for premature labour is controversial. The most likely treatment if you are less than thirty-four weeks pregnant is a drip containing a beta blocker (Betamimetic drug). If labour is not too advanced the drug will probably stop the contractions, though once the treatment has been stopped, its effects don't often last more than a week or so. However, this is long enough to allow for steroid treatment (by injection), which is said to hasten the maturity of the baby's lungs so that it will be better able to cope with breathing once it is delivered.

The combined treatment may well give a tiny premature baby a better start. However, neither of these drugs have been fully tested, and the beta blockers are known to have side effects on mothers suffering from heart diseases, high blood pressure and diabetes. Because of this uncertainty about the long-term effects of drugs some doctors avoid them and prefer to rely instead on the skill of paediatricians and staff in the special care baby unit.

Herpes virus

Herpes is the source both of cold sores and of a genital infection. It is the genital virus which is a problem during pregnancy.

Most herpes sufferers are only too aware of the condition. Painful blisters appear around the entrance to the vagina and they may get a slight fever too. These attacks can recur. The dangers of herpes is that the baby, on its way through the vagina, comes up against the open sores. Herpes is an extremely dangerous infection for a baby. It can cause brain damage which may well be fatal.

Some doctors recommend a Caesarean to any woman who has had herpes in the past. Others say that it is only the first attack which really counts, and a third view is that these women should be screened during the final weeks of pregnancy to see whether the virus is present. If no blisters appear it would, they believe, be safe to give birth naturally.

Linda and Colin have both been herpes sufferers for years. Appalled at the lack of information available, they decided to pay for a computer search for all written studies of herpes in pregnancy over the last five years. They received copies of over 200 articles. The results were contradictory.

'I really wanted to have a home birth but, when we had read all this, and the case histories of babies with herpes, I just didn't feel I had the right to risk it. I think if I had been in a place where they could screen me properly I might have had a natural birth, but here, even when I have clearly had a recurrence, the swabs have always been negative. So I didn't have much confidence in them. In the end I agreed to a Caesarean.'

If you have herpes, read *The Herpes Manual* (see page 201).

Weight loss

In the few days before labour it is quite normal for your weight to drop slightly. However, if your weight drops over a longer period than a week, it may be evidence that your placenta is not functioning as well as it should. Do make sure that you really have lost weight and that the difference is not due to a change in the scales you are weighed on. Read the sections on 'Movements' and 'Late for dates' below before agreeing to induction.

Reduction in movements

Your baby won't be kicking all the time, but if you feel that movements are slowing down, particularly if you have also lost a little weight or if the pregnancy has gone beyond its expected date, you may like to check for yourself.

Healthy babies should move at least ten times in twelve hours. Occasionally a healthy baby can move less frequently but, as a rule, once movements have slowed down this far, your baby will be safer out than in.

Check movements by choosing a time of day when you can be sure of at least six hours without too much to distract you. Then note each movement on a pad writing down the time of the fifth one. (Some hospitals provide kick charts to be filled in.) If you don't reach five in six hours, contact your doctor and ask if you can have your baby's heart monitored. Even if movements have stopped altogether there will still be time to save your baby but you must contact your doctor or clinic immediately as the baby would need to be delivered quickly.

Late for dates

Don't worry if your expected date of confinement has come and gone. Your baby is just as likely to arrive up to two weeks after that date.

In a small number of pregnancies the baby is not born before the ageing placenta starts to wear out. In this case the baby is safer born than trying to live off an ailing placenta.

If it were easy to check on the condition of the placenta then doctors and midwives could simply ensure that all genuinely post mature babies were induced. Unfortunately available tests are not very accurate, and doctors may advise induction on the basis of dates alone. This 'caution' can result in the induction of babies that are immature, more prone to chest infections, and may even have to spend their first days in special care.

Your dilemma is whether to go with mother nature (and risk post maturity) or with father medicine (and risk prematurity). If you are more than one week overdue, you can make some of your own checks: is the expected date of confinement correct according to your own calculations (see page 46)? is the baby moving normally (see above)? are you still gaining weight?

Then ask for the tests described below. If there is any evidence from all these checks that your baby is not doing as well as it should, then induction is probably a sensible option. If there is no evidence that anything is wrong you could wait a while, and see if nature will take its course. There are a few suggestions on page 111 for helping things along.

Pat and Dave were expecting their second child, by their calculation, in three weeks. The hospital disagreed:

'They said the baby was a week overdue and should be induced. We knew it wasn't because we had planned it, but there didn't seem to be much we could do. When they delivered her, she was premature and had to spend the first week in a special incubator. When they took her out she caught a cold, which turned to pneumonia. A month later she died.'

On the other hand, for Mandy's baby an induction could have been life-saving:

'the placenta had stopped functioning and had almost disintegrated. I was told afterwards that the baby would almost certainly have died had I not been induced that day.'

Light for dates (small for dates)

A baby which seems to be smaller than it should be by the calculated age of pregnancy can also cause worry. If the baby really is too small it would be evidence that it is not getting enough nourishment from the placenta. This may mean that the placenta is failing. All the tests suggested for 'late for dates' babies would be used to try and work out whether the baby really is abnormally small, or just a small baby. Once again, you may well be the best judge of your baby's wellbeing and it is important to pay attention to its movements (see kick charts on page 95). If the baby really is not thriving inside it would be better out.

HOW TECHNOLOGY CAN HELP

Electronic heart monitoring

This will be done regularly if you are in hospital and can be done on an outpatient basis if there is any reason to believe that your baby is unwell.

Two straps will be fastened around your tummy. The upper one records any contractions you may have and the lower one picks up the baby's heartbeat. The two monitors are linked to a machine with a printed paper readout. There may also be a video screen on the monitor. The video patterns are very hard to follow and are best ignored.

What the machine means

A healthy heartbeat has a jagged, irregular rhythm. If the ups and downs start to smooth out your baby may be tiring. (It could also be a malfunction in the machine and that should be double checked.) The most important sign is a heartbeat pattern that dips. (See illustration on page 98.) *If you are in labour* and the dips occur as you contract and go up again immediately afterwards there is probably no problem but the medical staff should be vigilant. These are called type 1 dips. If the dips come in between contractions (type 2 as they are known) it is a clear sign of foetal distress and shouldn't be ignored.

The monitor will also have a scale, or a flashing number indicating the number of heartbeats per minute (HPM). This would normally register somewhere between 120 and 160. The staff are watching for a variation of more than twenty beats either way.

Drawbacks of electronic monitoring

If the machine isn't working properly, or the people minding it do not know how to interpret an unusual reading, you may get a false alarm. It is not unknown for a Caesarean section to be performed on the basis of a faulty monitor. On the other hand there have recently been cases where staff have ignored signs of real distress, because they had become so used to machines that don't work properly.

Any changes should be gradual. Sudden changes are likely to be electrical faults or the effect of the baby turning away from

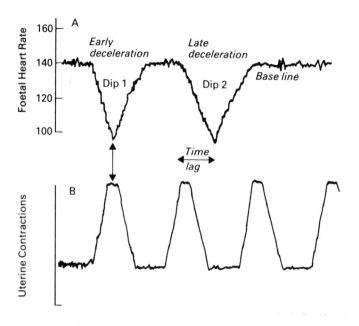

Foetal heart monitoring charts showing relationship between uterine contractions and foetal heart rate, early sounds (*Aberdeen Maternity Hospital*)

Type 1 Dips: the baby's heart rate slows with each contraction. This is not serious but should be watched.

Type 2 Dips: the baby's heart rate slows between contractions. This is more serious and you should call for a midwife immediately.

the monitor. So if the heart noise stops, or the line suddenly flattens, ask for a double check with a portable sonic aid (midwives' listening device) – the belt may need moving or you may get another machine. If the trace is showing clear dips unassociated with contractions, don't wait to double check, your baby's life may be in danger. It should be delivered as soon as possible, usually by Caesarean.

Placental function tests

These can give some information about the baby's health. They are:

Human placental lactogen (HPL) tests which are carried out on a blood sample; or

Oestriol tests which check the level of the hormone oestrogen in your urine.

A healthy placenta should give out an increasing amount of hormone as pregnancy progresses, which drops off just before the start of labour. Unfortunately doctors can only test the hormone that the placenta is getting rid of, which is not a very accurate way of finding out what it is using.

Your oestrogen level changes all the time. The test must show if it is actually dropping, so you will need a series of blood or urine tests over a number of days if the information is to be at all useful. (You may be asked to collect all your urine for twenty-four hours, though more modern tests do not require this.) A low hormone level is probably not as important as a level which is clearly going down.

As these tests tend to overestimate problems by quite a large percentage, they should really be looked at alongside a kick chart.

Ultrasound scanning (see page 67) may be useful now if you have had base line scans earlier in pregnancy. It can show whether the baby is growing steadily.

Kick charts are probably the most reliable monitors and you can do these yourself (see page 95).

Continuity of care Probably the best check of all is a competent midwife who has seen you through pregnancy, and can judge by feel, and with a tape measure, the gradual growth of your tummy and your baby. Sadly few of us are blessed with such individual attention.

Induction

Induction (when labour is started artificially) now happens in over 25 per cent of pregnancies. (It seems unlikely that nature can be wrong as often as this.) Here is a list of the possible reasons why the doctors may suggest induction.

High blood pressure because of its effects on the placenta and mother (see page 86)

Post maturity

Small pelvis or large baby (page 92)
Diabetes
Small for dates (page 96)

It is also done for other severe complications such as Rhesus haemolytic disease or certain foetal abnormalities. If your baby dies in the womb, induction would be performed to deliver it as soon as possible, and spare you any more distress.

Disadvantages of induction

1 If the induction is performed before the baby is mature there is greater risk of chest infections, breathing difficulties, and transfer to a special care baby unit after the birth.
2 Many women who have experienced both a natural and an induced labour say that an induced labour is more painful and harder to cope with without drugs.
3 There is more chance of medical intervention; electronic monitoring will be necessary to regulate the rate of induction (which restricts movement); stronger painkillers may be required (see page 131); you may then need a forceps delivery and this would mean a large cut (episiotomy) to help the baby out. Of course this chain of events doesn't always occur and if you need the induction for the sake of the baby you would probably be prepared to put up with everything else anyway.
4 Occasionally induction may fail and labour stops. If this happens, you could end up needing a Caesarean. This happens less when Prostaglandin Jel is used to soften the cervix the night before the drip is set up.
5 In a small number of cases, induction has been known to cause contractions which are so strong they damage the womb.
6 There seems also to be some evidence of an increase in excessive bleeding after delivery which cannot then be stopped by the administration of more oxytocic drugs (see page 137).
7 Some studies show a small increase in foetal distress and respiratory problems in babies. This may be due to the stronger contractions cutting the oxygen supply to the placenta.
8 There is more risk of neonatal jaundice.

According to the *British Way of Birth*, the BBC Television survey, women who were induced were mostly unhappy about the procedure even though 10 per cent who filled in the questionnaire had asked for induction. For more on induction, see page 136.

Caesarean section

An operation to deliver the baby may be planned in the following situations:

1 Small pelvis/large baby (see page 92)
2 Placenta praevia (see page 90)
3 Breech presentation, or if the baby is stuck in a position which would make ordinary delivery impossible.
4 Foetal distress, when there is evidence before labour starts that the baby's heartbeat is not normal.
5 If you have an active case of genital herpes (HSV).
6 When the baby needs to be delivered early but induction is impractical.

In all these cases, a Caesarean will be planned in advance of the start of labour, or as a possible option after a 'trial of labour'. In some hospitals, Caesareans can be done using *epidural* anaesthesia (see page 131). An epidural is safer than a general anaesthetic both for you and the baby so it is worth asking for. As a herpes sufferer, Linda asked for an epidural Caesarean.

'They put a screen up so that we couldn't actually see what they were doing. I could feel it but there was absolutely no pain. My baby was given to me to hold five minutes later and I held her while they stitched me up. It was a really good experience.'

It may seem like a relief to do away with the pain of labour but a Caesarean is still a major abdominal operation and should never be carried out unless a vaginal delivery would clearly be dangerous to you or the baby.

Once you have had one Caesarean there is a risk that future babies would also have to be delivered that way and, with a scar on your womb, you would be considered a relatively high risk in future pregnancies.

Oddly enough babies seem to find the sudden delivery more

of a shock than a vaginal delivery and may be slower to breathe and suck.

In spite of these drawbacks, Caesareans are very safe these days, so if you find that you need one you can look forward to it with confidence (see page 142 for more on Caesareans).

PREPARATION FOR PARENTHOOD

Leaving work

With your first pregnancy the few weeks between leaving work and becoming a mother can seem very empty. Anne Oakley interviewed women about their feelings at this time: Tanya Kemp had a busy, responsible job as a medical receptionist. She said,

> 'You feel so useless. Whereas at work you've always got people depending on you all the time, decisions to make. Now I'm hoovering, dusting, doing all the housework – which doesn't take long. I feel lost.'

On the other hand, if your job was physically demanding, you may be more than ready for a rest. Nina Brady was a shop assistant but she had to give that up earlier in pregnancy because her legs ached. She got another job and had to give that up because of the heat:

> 'There was a week there, in August, that was very hot. I collapsed, had to give it up. I get very tired when I wash a few cups – I get killed out . . . I spend most of my time in bed.'

The enforced idleness of late pregnancy can breed anxiety. Lois said,

> 'I was vaguely thinking, I've got another ten or twelve weeks until I go back to work and then yesterday it suddenly occurred to me for the first time that I can't think in terms of ten or twelve weeks because I'm going to have a baby for the last seven weeks of that. I think I panicked for the first time in my pregnancy. It did really occur to me that I was going to have responsibility towards something . . . then I started thinking, what are all the other things that I should be fitting

into these next six weeks? Because it's the last time in my life I'm going to have six weeks free.'

Organising your home

'If anyone in our house got a nesting instinct it was John. While I made a baby, he made cupboards, decorated and tried to turn our tiny flat into a place suitable for a child.'

Heat
You should have at least one room which can be kept at a constant temperature of 68° day and night. Even if you have central heating, unless your baby is born in midsummer you may need extra heating during the night.

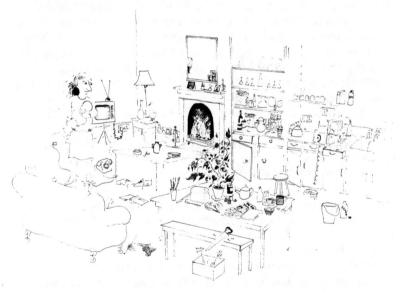

In next to no time your baby will be crawling. . . . You would do well to start clearing every breakable object.

Space
In next to no time your baby will be crawling, and before you have got used to that, she'll be pulling herself up on your book-

shelves to investigate your most precious objects. While you still have time you would do well to start clearing every breakable object at least three feet above floor level. Kiss goodbye to your glass coffee table with lethal corners, and any other objects and obstructions which could prove hazardous to a newly staggering child somewhere at knee level.

Cupboards fixed high up on the wall or fitted with childproof catches will save you endless battles of will and protect your china. A large, floor-level cupboard into which toys can be unceremoniously swept at the end of the day is a great help when you want to create a few child-free moments in the evening. If you are redecorating, or buying new furniture, stick to washable paint (wallpaper is a joy to pick off) and avoid light, plain fabrics and carpets unless you want to spend a fortune on cleaning.

Equipment

Keep an eye on local paper small ads, newsagents' windows, clinic noticeboards and, of course, friends and relations for secondhand bargains. Baby equipment can circulate for years before it wears out. It is worth making sure that the equipment on offer is really the most useful design for you. A large carriage-sprung pram will do nothing but clutter your hall, unless your front door opens directly on to the street.

An automatic washing machine is the most useful piece of equipment money can buy. If the choice is between a cot and a pram or a washing machine, buy the washing machine. You will never regret it.

Somewhere to sleep for the early weeks is really no problem. Some people like to have their babies in bed with them. Otherwise, a carrycot, a Moses basket, or even a large cardboard box with a mattress will do, as long as the baby is warm. A drop side cot won't be necessary for about six months. If you do put a small baby in a big cot it is safer to use a 'bumper'.

Baby nests which are padded with drawstrings round the top are no longer considered safe for tiny babies. Pillows are not safe either. A baby who is too small to turn its head may well suffocate on the folds of material. Your 'cot' should have a firm, smooth mattress with no obstructions around the face. Cellular blankets are best. They are light, warm and full of holes. The baby should have no trouble breathing even if the covers do go over her head.

A baby sling is the simplest solution in the early weeks. Make sure it supports the baby's neck and head and distributes the weight evenly across your back and shoulders to prevent backache. Babies love this method of transport and will snuggle up and sleep happily. They are also a godsend at night for quietening a restless, wakeful baby.

Prams are best for parents who travel mostly on foot and in the immediate area. Look for one which has a back rest and rings for a safety harness so that it will still be useful when your baby is sitting up. Some prams fold down to become pushchairs in later life.

Convertibles are a better solution for those living above ground level. MacLaren do a carrycot frame which converts to a foldaway 'buggy' pushchair. The carrycot is a bit small to take a large baby right through to the sitting-up stage, so, if big babies run in the family, you would be better off with more specialised equipment.

Carrycots are essential for car travellers. You should also buy a safety harness to hold it safely in place on the back seat. If you buy a set of wheels to go under it you will be fully equipped for travelling, walking and sleeping for the first six months. Again, it pays to buy the longest cot you can with a back rest and safety rings so that your baby can use it until she is old enough to be strapped into a car baby seat at about six months.

Lie back buggies are the most convenient solution if you expect to have to carry the whole contraption, plus baby, up and down stairs and on and off buses. There are several different models which recline so that a tiny baby can travel lying down. You can then convert it to an upright buggy later on. Look for a model which is comfortable to push and doesn't give you a backache.

Bathing can be managed in the kitchen sink if your kitchen can be made warm enough. If this isn't practical, you will feel safest with a baby bath which is sloped at one end so that the baby cannot go under (in the unlikely event that you might drop her). You can of course bath your baby with you, but don't make the water too hot.

Covering bottoms
This is the subject of fierce advertising controversy. There are basically three kinds of nappies: terry towelling, disposable pads with separate plastic pants, and expensive all-in-wonderful dis-

posables. There is no real cost difference between the first two but the all-in-ones are more expensive. Some parents use terries for the early weeks, and later for night, and disposables during the day.

Disposables   Tiny babies are better covered with pads. The all-in-ones, even with elastic legs, are not much good at keeping things in. Tie plastic pants can more easily be adjusted to the individual (see page 172). Pads with water-resistant covers, which don't disintegrate so easily, such as 'Bambis' may be more comfortable for the baby, though they are a little more expensive.

For older babies all-in-one nappies are almost as wonderful as the ads suggest. However, there is no evidence that your baby will cry any less in them! Even if you are a convinced terry user, a pack of all-in-ones is a useful back-up for journeys, and days when you feel like a rest. Shop around for bargains. Chain stores are rarely the cheapest stockists.

Terry towelling   Terry users need washing machines if they are to avoid constant drudgery. Terry nappies are very absorbent, less likely to leak and, combined with one-way liners (disposable by day and fabric by night), are not too hard on bottoms. Look out for 'seconds' of good brands. Two dozen thick nappies may (just) see you through two babies. You will also need a couple of buckets with lids and some steriliser (you can use ordinary household bleach). Fabric softener can cause a rash so use it cautiously. Tie plastic pants can be used to cover terries as well as pads (see page 172). They are cheap, adjustable, less likely than most pants to go hard and stiff and they dry more easily.

Clothing tips for the baby

For some reason, most books advise you to get four pairs of stretch suits for a new baby. Since it is not unusual for a baby to go through that number in a day you may well find you need more. You will have enough on your mind in the early weeks without worrying whether you have anything to clothe the baby in while you are washing the garment which she has just wet, or been sick on. So try not to let pride stand in the way of accepting hand-me-downs or scouring jumble sales. The less you spend on first-size clothes, the better. They will only last three months at the most.

Warmth is important. Stretch suits keep everything covered no matter how much she kicks and wriggles. A nightie may seem more convenient for night nappy changing, but a wriggly baby may kick it up and get cold. A dressing gown with buttons at the bottom is ideal for winter. You will also need vests, a couple of cardigans, bootees and mittens and a woolly hat. A large woollen shawl can replace all this in the first few weeks but it doesn't allow much freedom for kicking.

Avoid stretchsuits that are taken on and off over the head (not a pleasant job if they get dirty); small head holes (look for poppers or buttons on the shoulder instead); ribbons or tapes which are dangerous; thin cotton dresses which are unlikely to be warm enough for a young baby; and white woollies which will need constant washing.

Toiletries for babies are overrated and overpriced. You need:
1 a mild baby soap for washing at bath time and nappy changes;
2 a large tub of zinc and castor oil (though some babies are allergic to this) or Vaseline, for waterproofing the baby's bottom;
3 cotton wool;
4 baby bubble bath which can replace soap and is less slippery if you are a bit nervous.

You do not need:
1 baby wipes and baby lotion which can irritate sensitive skin;
2 talcum powder, which could be inhaled, possibly damaging your baby's lungs.

You can manage without:
1 a changing mat – though it is usefully easy to clean;
2 a special changing bag – a plastic bag makes a perfectly good container for travelling.

COUNTDOWN TO THE BIRTH

'After weeks of exhaustion I suddenly felt full of energy and rushed off to the art galleries that I wouldn't have time to visit for a long time afterwards.'

Checklist for labour

1 Put the telephone number of your midwife, or hospital near the phone where you can find it in a hurry.
2 If you don't have a phone have you asked a neighbour if you can borrow theirs, or checked that the nearest call box actually works?
3 Have you made plans for a friend to care for any other children during labour?
4 Can you contact your partner, or labour companion, easily? Do you know exactly where he or she will be in the next few days?
5 Check what your hospital procedure is and write it down.
6 Pack your bag to avoid forgetting important things in the rush.
7 Check with your midwife what you will need to provide if you are having a home birth.

Supplies for labour

1 Glucose or dextrose tablets in case you get tired and need a boost. (They go down easily and may help you avoid a drip in a long labour.)
2 An ice pack, hot water bottle, and couple of tennis balls in a sock! (If you have a backache labour (see page 128) they could be a great comfort.)
3 A sponge for mopping your brow and occasional sips of water.
4 If you are going by car, some extra cushions to prop you up during the birth.
5 Your companion's food and drink (hospital canteens don't operate round the clock).
6 A camera, with film in it, to record the occasion.
7 A notebook and pen for your birth record (to be kept by your companion).
8 Warm socks and a shawl or cardigan in case you get the shivers.

For the hospital

1 At least two nighties which unbutton in the front for breast-feeding and a dressing gown (hospitals usually insist that you are 'decently' covered).
2 Money for the telephone (plenty of it) and phone numbers of friends and relations.
3 Earplugs (wax ones available from Boots) to block out the sound of other people's babies. You can hear your own through reinforced concrete.
4 Disposable knickers to save yourself washing. You probably won't need a sanitary belt. You can put the pads in your knickers.
5 Soft lavatory paper which hospitals, for some reason, don't supply in maternity wards.
6 A bag of bran to add to every meal (no one wants to be constipated when they've got stitches).
7 A child's rubber ring which will make sitting easier if you have stitches.
8 A nipple spray (such as Rotersept) in case you get sore nipples.
9 Comfrey ointment (from a chemist which sells herbal medicines). It is very soothing if you have stitches.
10 This book.

Chapter 5

LABOUR

WHAT IS LABOUR?

'I feel no pain, just a massive strong muscle in the centre of my whole being working intensely hard towards the birth.'

During labour the criss-cross bands of muscle in your uterus start to work, triggered by a hormone (oxytoxin). Usually they start quite gently in widely spaced waves getting stronger and more intense as labour progresses. Some women go straight into intense contractions which are quite close together.

In the *first stage* of labour the womb muscles are thickening at the top and pushing the baby's head down. The long vertical muscles are also working, pulling the neck of the womb (*cervix*) up and outwards.

The *second stage* starts when the cervix is fully open (*dilated*). The round muscles start squeezing in and out to push the baby out.

The *third stage* comes after the birth when the *placenta*, which has nourished the baby in the womb, is expelled.

Does it hurt?

There is a theory that muscles contracting cannot hurt and pain only occurs if you tense up and your body works against the contractions producing a 'tug of war'. It seems to be true that approaching labour in an optimistic frame of mind, welcoming and accepting the strong sensations, goes a long way towards a good labour. However we do not believe that pain is simply a symptom of fear. In fact, if you are led to believe that it won't hurt, the shock of strong contractions may themselves cause you to lose control and make matters worse.

All of us who were directly involved in writing this book

felt pain during labour. We felt it in varying degrees and coped in different ways. We don't believe that you can banish pain simply by learning your lessons well. But we do believe that your memories of your baby's birth can, like ours, number amongst the happiest of your life, even if your labour does not work out as you expected.

Getting things started

If your date of delivery has come and gone there are some things you can do to get things started. None of these methods will work if your body, and your baby, are not ready for labour so don't worry about triggering a premature labour.

Breast stimulation releases natural oxytocin in your body. You may notice when you breastfeed your baby that the sucking causes mild cramps as it helps you pull your womb back into shape. Sucking, stroking, or whatever feels good can produce the same effect before the baby is born, and may get your labour started.

Orgasm makes your womb contract and this can also be a useful nudge to your system.

Prostaglandin is found naturally in semen. If you make love, your partner's ejaculate contains as much prostaglandin as some tablets or pessaries used to soften the cervix and to help dilate it.

Castor oil cocktail is an old remedy for starting labour. It works, like an enema, to clean out your system and the action can trigger off muscle action in your womb. Since castor oil tastes rather unpleasant try this recipe to make it more palatable: 1 inch of orange juice in a glass, 2–3 tablespoons of castor oil and 2 heaped teaspoons of Andrews Liver Salts. Drink it immediately while it is still frothy.

THE STAGES OF LABOUR

The start

Here are a few descriptions of the start of labour.

* *'They were every eight minutes, a strong alternating with a weak. Not at all painful, rather like ripples inside.'*

* 'Had a show [see below] at midday and went for a longish walk. Contractions were hourly. By 6 p.m. they were every 15 minutes or so. By 8.20 they were coming every 7–8 minutes in the back like mild period pains.'
* 'I felt a funny movement rather like a bubble of air in my back and I realised that the waters had gone.'
* 'My waters leaked all day, I had a show, went in at 10 p.m. and had Sophie at 11.55. I must admit that deep inside I felt a little panic.'
* 'Expected day of delivery – cleaned the cooker. That should have told me something as it's the first time for months.'
* 'Thursday was the big day. I had loads of energy and felt fine. I did all the housework, bathed the dog and didn't have time for a rest that afternoon. I went out in the evening and got home about 12.30. I wasn't even tired. My waters went as soon as I got into bed. I was so pleased that something positive was happening all I could do was laugh.'

Women often fear that they will miss the early signs of labour and give birth on a bus. It is actually far more likely that you will go too early into hospital and spend many boring hours in a strange environment when you could have been coping perfectly well at home. These are the likely early signs of labour:

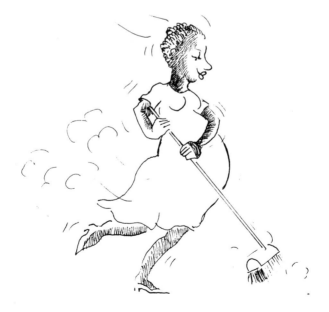

1 Your weight may drop a few days before labour is due.
2 A sudden surge of energy in the last day or so is very common.
3 Diarrhoea may precede labour by a few hours (nature's enema).
4 A small quantity of mucus which is usually blood-stained may come away anything up to a week before the labour. It is called the 'show'. (It is a very small amount of blood, bleeding severe enough to warrant the use of a second pad should be reported immediately to your doctor.)
5 Low backache, like a period pain, may herald the start of regular contractions.
6 Light contractions, when your tummy goes hard and square shaped, start coming every half hour or so. You don't need to go into hospital until they are coming roughly every three to five minutes and lasting fifty seconds, or feel strong enough to stop you doing anything else.

   If you live a fair distance from the hospital you will have to take that into account and start your journey before they become too intense. As sitting may be uncomfortable during contractions it helps to travel in the back so that you can get down on all fours if necessary. If you are having a home birth or 'domino' delivery you should contact your midwife as soon as contractions become regular so that she can plan her day.
7 The bag of waters, in which the baby is floating, may burst at the start of labour. It may leak out in a dribble or gush out in a warm flood which needs a towel to soak it up.

   Contractions usually start soon after but they may be delayed. In nearly all cases they start within twenty-four hours.

   If your baby is not yet due, or does not have its head well down in the pelvis, a midwife should check that the cord has not prolapsed (come down in front of the baby's head) as this would be dangerous for the baby.

   If you know that the baby's head is engaged (look on your Coop card) there is really no rush to go into hospital. They may want to induce contractions to speed labour in case of infection. If you are not keen to be induced you can safely wait for twelve hours or more without risk to the baby. You could use the time at home trying the suggestions on page

111 to get your labour going. Do, however, avoid bathing or making love which could introduce infection.

The first stage

'7 a.m., I can feel the muscle pulling upwards and stretching. It is very easy to ride using slow, deliberate breathing, very calm and deep. I've had ten hours' sleep and I feel good.

I get up and carry on as usual just stopping to squat with each contraction. They are coming every ten minutes now, for thirty seconds.

I go for a pee every hour. This not only makes me feel better, it speeds up the labour too. It must be the walking, I wish I felt like moving around more.

The contractions continue in the same pattern but they are getting much stronger. I'm using mouth-centred [see page 126] breathing now. It is hard work but I am enjoying myself.

2.30 – an internal examination. I am half dilated now and the contractions are very strong. I use distraction words [see page 127] with them all. Disappear is a good one. It makes me concentrate just enough to keep on top of the contractions.

At 3.20 I am fully dilated.'

What is happening?

During the first stage of labour the muscles of the womb are contracting and expanding to stretch the neck of the womb to its limit (about 10cms or five fingers). This stage can last one hour or twenty-four hours. In a first labour it will probably be between eight and twelve hours. Other labours are usually shorter.

A long labour need not be a bad labour. The contractions may be spaced out and quite gentle for most of it and, as Marie remarked,

'Time feels different in labour. It did drag on a bit but it certainly didn't feel like twenty-four hours to me.'

A short labour, on the other hand, may not always be a good one. The contractions may be very close together and intense, right from the start, which can be a bit of a shock to the system. In some cases, a short labour seems short just because most of the first stage has been painless and you do not actually notice contractions until your cervix is wide open and you are ready to push the baby out.

How can you help yourself?

Eat lightly early on as it may be a long time until your next meal and you will need plenty of energy to see you through. As labour progresses you can sip fruit juice (avoid orange or grapefruit which are acidic) or eat glucose tablets to give you the occasional energy boost (a better way of keeping up your strength than a glucose drip).

Keep upright, and moving around, for as long as you feel comfortable. This will speed contractions, make them more efficient, and keep up the blood flow to your baby. It helps to have a strong piece of furniture to lean on during contractions. Squatting during contractions may also feel comfortable.

If this sounds too strenuous, it is better to sit, rather than to lie down. The baby is being pushed downwards and if you sit, or squat, you will be adding the force of gravity to the force of contractions. If your womb is having to push the baby up and along it will need far more energy to do it. If you are upright you will get almost twice as much work out of every contraction.

If the pain is felt mainly in your back, your baby may be lying in the posterior position (see page 82). Going on all fours may take some of the strain off your back. As your vagina is angled slightly forwards this is a better position than lying flat on your back.

Of course you may feel that you just have to lie down. In this case, lie on your side, or well propped up with cushions to keep the pressure off the big arteries running up your back which are carrying blood to your baby.

A warm bath is usually a great comfort. If the water can be kept warm and the bath full it takes the pressure off your body and will help you relax. Robyn liked the bath so much that she ended up having her baby in it:

'I went to have a bath to see if it would relax me. It felt better because I could move more easily. My husband and Melody [her midwife] took turns rocking me. I was in there five hours. Once in I didn't want to get out.'

Pee regularly every hour (get your partner to remind you). This ensures that your bladder is empty and isn't obstructing the baby. It also gives you a reason to get up and move around which will speed your labour.

Notes for your companion
Once labour has started most other things will be wiped out of your partner's mind. Read the lists on page 108 and make sure everything is prepared.

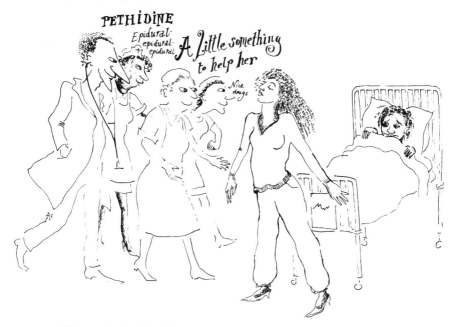

Your role in the labour will depend very much on the attitude of the staff. At home you will have rather more freedom. Many midwives these days will be happy to have you there and recognise your importance as a comforter, morale booster and interpreter of hospital procedure and suggested treatment. Others may see you as a threat and treat you as such. Nina was a companion to her friend Rita:

'I suspected that I would have to act as a protective shield and I felt that I was being so. The midwife suggested that Rita should have "something to help her" after her bath. I asked her what she meant, to be absolutely clear about it, and said that we wanted to manage without pethidine if possible. It felt as though a battle had begun.'

Massage may help especially if the pain is in her back. Don't scrub at her, massage slowly or simply apply pressure. Some childbirth teachers recommend a long sock with two tennis balls in it to roll up and down her back, or for her to lean against. Play this by ear. Some women find they cannot bear to be touched during labour.

Relaxation between contractions is important. Touch, stroke, or point to, the tensed up muscles to remind her to relax them.

Timing contractions will give you a clearer sense of the progress of labour if you are not using a monitor. Time from the beginning of one contraction to the beginning of the next and the length of the contraction itself. This information will be useful if she decides to use gas and air (see page 128).

Transition

Jennie felt

'completely isolated by the need to concentrate on the contractions. I imagined a mountain sitting on my belly with the arrival of each contraction. I imagined myself walking up a downward escalator so ensuring that I never reached the top until the contraction was over. I repeated to myself: "you're climbing up the mountain and you are going to reach the top very soon." '

What is happening?
Your cervix is nearly fully open now with just one, or two centimetres to go. The pattern of contractions will start to change as the womb gets ready to push the baby down. These contractions can be very strong and confusing, sometimes you will get double peaks to each one, or they may come very close together. It is the hardest part of the labour for those women who experience it (some don't) and it can last for a few minutes to an hour, occasionally longer.

Anthea describes feeling

'a bit desperate. I didn't know which bloody level I was breathing in and I didn't care. I said all the things I was told I would say: "I want to go home," "I want to rest," "I don't want a baby," "I can't go on any more." I could hear myself

saying it and I thought: "I suppose this is transition, well I don't want it." I didn't want anything except oblivion.'

The signs of transition may be: an attack of the shakes, vomiting, feeling hot and cold, and a feeling of pressure against your lower back and bottom. You may feel angry, despondent and weepy and demand pain relief, thinking 'sod the baby what about me?' If you know this is transition you may feel able to wait until it is over and manage without drugs, but if you can't, don't feel you've failed, you are in good company.

How can you help yourself?

Concentrate on your body and treat each contraction as if it were the only one. If one of them overwhelms you, put it behind you and concentrate on the next one. Try to see each new contraction as a welcome step towards the end of labour.

Controlling the urge to push may be the biggest frustration of all. If you push too soon, the baby's head may bruise the cervix, causing swelling. Then transition can take longer.

Sometimes, particularly if you have been lying down, the cervix hasn't opened quite evenly and you have what the midwives will call an '*anterior lip*' of cervix which hasn't stretched completely. The midwife may be able to push it over the baby's head during a contraction. Until the cervix is wide open, the best thing you can do is the 'hoo ha ha' breathing mentioned on page 127 which will stop you getting enough air in your lungs for a good push.

Notes for your companion

The most obvious outward sign of transition is the emotional change that usually accompanies it. The sheer intensity of the contractions may cause a usually calm and cheerful person to swear and curse, cry out and generally lose all her inhibitions. Yes, it probably does hurt, but you won't help if you burst into tears in sympathy. Try not to leave the room at all during this phase, you will be sorely missed. Help her to get her breathing back into order when she loses track; if she feels the urge to push, call a midwife and ask her to check the cervix. The knowledge that the baby is nearly there is the best news you can convey.

John said,

'I was very apprehensive. The baby seemed to have stopped

*moving and you seemed very tired. I was already starting to
feel quite strained. It was difficult to appreciate that you
needed me because you seemed so far away. But you clearly
did need me. You didn't want me to leave the room. The
midwife, who hadn't spoken to me till then, made it clear that
she appreciated the role I was playing, comforting you.'*

It can be a great help to tap or clap out the rhythm of breathing,
as Phil did:

*'Phil did some back massage but I couldn't bear to be touched.
I needed to be able to see him so that we could breathe
together. He would say: "open your eyes, look at me, come on,
puff, puff, blow." He really kept me going.'*

If your partner wants to stand, she will need support during the
contractions. You can hold her as though you were dancing, or
support her with your arms around her from behind.

Second stage

*'I did a lot of shouting, not pushing. Somehow my body didn't
seem to require help. It was pushing without my consciously
helping it other than by shouting. It seemed odd that they
were saying "well done, that's a good one", when I wasn't
doing anything. The noise helped, it really did. At one stage it
sounded as though it came from elsewhere. I felt grateful to it
because it helped me. I remember appealing to the babe to
hurry up and get born.'*

What is happening?
Your cervix is now as wide as it can be and the muscles in your
womb start the job of pushing the baby down through the vagina.
For some women this is the best part of labour:

*'Second stage lasted forty-five minutes and it was fantastic. I
really got into the pushing technique and enjoyed every
minute, getting five good pushes with every contraction.'*

Others disagree:

*'At no time did I think the urge to push at all wonderful. It
just felt like something that I had to do as quickly as possible.'*

How can you help yourself?

Your position during this stage is important. If you have the energy and inclination, you could try kneeling, squatting or on all fours. This is easier on the floor, but if you are on a bed it helps if two people can support you. In these positions your bottom is off the bed so the coccyx (the end of your spine) can move back slightly out of the way of the head.

Some midwives are rather alarmed at the idea of delivering in these positions but it is worth remembering that the majority of the world's babies arrive with the help of gravity.

Pushing   In this country the normal style in second stage is to encourage the woman to take a deep breath, hold it, and then push like mad. Some recent studies indicate that babies are better off if their mothers push according to the demands of their own bodies with several short pushes to each contraction.

Your womb will do most of the work by itself. Try not to hold your breath for very long because you will be cutting off your baby's supply of oxygen temporarily.

Some women are overwhelmed by the urge to push. If you are not, you don't have to put on a good show. Just try and work with your body rather than against it.

It sometimes helps to fix your mind on a spot on the wall and then aim to push the baby out towards it. Alternatively, if someone can hold a mirror up for you so that you can see your baby's head bobbing backwards and forwards with each push, you can mentally aim towards the mirror.

Relaxing your vagina while you are pushing may seem impossible. But try to do it because the muscles there, though elastic, are strong and you want them to relax and let your baby through. It may help to picture your vagina and imagine the folds of flesh unfurling like pleats.

Notes for your companion

'There was no time to talk to Leslie but I was glad he was there. He suggested that I got into a sitting position. It seemed too much trouble at the time. I wish that he and the doctor had agreed it would help and moved me up the bed. As it was, the pillows were too far back to support me and I delivered flat on my back.'

You can do a great deal to help now. Suggest a different posture, perhaps one you have already practised, and then help her into the right position. If she is too tired to move very much by herself, you can pull her back up the bed between contractions and pile the pillows up, or sit behind her yourself so that she is supported against you. Remember that it really is easier to give birth propped up and help accordingly. It's much easier to squat if you are on a mattress on the floor. In some hospitals this can be easily arranged and it's certainly a good idea at home. Some hospitals are also acquiring birthing stools and chairs to help in second stage. Find out in advance if any of these things can be used.

The birth

'I pushed like mad and felt this stretching, burning feeling. I was told to pant and, though I couldn't really stop pushing, I did try a bit. Then they put my hands round the baby's head and, as I pushed, I felt the slithery body oozing out of me. I dumped it on my tummy, rolled it over, and opened my eyes. It was a third boy.'

What is happening?

As the baby's head stretches the vaginal opening wide (this is called *crowning*) you will feel a strange stretching feeling which one woman described as like 'splitting in half'. (If you want to know what this feels like try stretching your mouth as wide as you can with two fingers in the corners. That is very much like the feeling of crowning.) If you put your hands down and touch the baby's head you may be reassured to discover that it is smaller than it feels.

If the vaginal opening looks likely to tear the midwife may decide to cut it (see *episiotomy*, page 140) to help the baby out. Once the head is born, she will check with her fingers to see whether the cord is round the neck (it will be in one birth out of every three), in which case she will either have to cut it, or pull it over the head.

In some hospitals it is routine practice to stick a tube up the baby's nose and into its mouth in order to clear any mucus out of the passages to the lungs. This is important only if the baby's breathing is being obstructed. If you would rather the midwife avoided the procedure until it is clearly necessary, make your feelings known in advance.

Once the head is out, the midwife will support it as it turns to allow the shoulders and body to slide out, often accompanied by a noise which John described as 'like the water draining out of the bath'.

The moment of birth may be more exciting for your companion than for you. I wrote at the time,

'Finally he burst out, blinked and looked around. The relief was exquisite.'

Nina, who helped her friend through labour, wrote,

'The actual appearance of that little head was marvellous. It was euphoric.'

Helping yourself

As the baby crowns, the midwife will ask you to stop pushing and pant, to stop the baby shooting out and hitting the wall. Pant slowly and gently, at the same time letting your jaw sag. If your mouth is relaxed it will help you to relax your vaginal and pelvic floor muscles, allowing the tissue to stretch just that little bit extra.

You might like to put your hands down and slide them under your baby's arms delivering her or him on to your own tummy. This is possible even if you end up needing a cut and forceps to help the baby out (see page 141) and it is a very good way to start life.

How your companion can help

If you can manage it, this is of course the moment to take that photograph, if you cannot no one will ever blame you. Just being there is what matters:

'I remembered to look, it was amazing. A real baby of our own all blood with a cord and all. We could see it was a girl and Dave suddenly hugged me just as if I'd scored a goal.'

The first moments together

It helps to wear a front opening gown or your partner can help you pull your gown right back just before the birth so that you really feel that hot little body in direct contact with yours.

Once you have greeted your baby, in most hospitals, the cord will be cut and the baby whipped away to be wrapped. It is very important to keep the baby warm. Their heat regulating mechanisms are not yet working properly and they can very easily get chilled. However, it is perfectly possible for a blanket to be laid over both of you (women often feel very chilly themselves immediately after labour), so that your baby can experience the comfort and warmth of your body and hear the beating of your heart while adjusting to this strange new world.

Suckling

If you intend to breastfeed your baby it helps to start as soon as possible (see page 160). The effect of the sucking will also release oxytocin into your bloodstream which will help your uterus to contract, expelling the placenta (if it hasn't already been removed) and closing off the blood vessels in your womb.

Checking your baby's health

As soon as your baby is born, the midwife will make a quick visual check of its condition which she will later record as an APGAR score. Usually if the 'score' is less than 3/10 at one minute or 5/10 at five minutes a paediatrician (baby specialist) will be called.

Five signs are checked and your baby will get either 0, 1 or 2 for each indication. They are:

1 *Colour*: at birth your baby will be pale blue or mauvish. As he or she starts to breathe, the colour will change. White-skinned babies start to look pink within about five minutes though the legs and arms may remain bluish for a little longer. Black babies can start life looking very pale but don't worry, the darker colour comes in over the first few days, though it can take longer for the full skin colour to come in.

2 *Respiratory effort* (breathing) is usually judged by the amount of noise your baby makes. Of course a baby which is handled very gently at birth may not make a great deal of noise and yet still be breathing regularly and strongly. The old-fashioned slap on the back is not necessary.

3 *Heartbeat* is measured. If it is over 100 the baby gets two points. Less than that only one point is awarded and if there is no heartbeat some action would be taken immediately.

4 *Muscle tone* is checked. If the baby is moving actively it will get two points.

5 *Response to stimulation* is also scored. If the baby cries at its

first experience of life then that is a definite response to stimulation.

Resuscitation If your baby does not start to breathe straight away you may be alarmed by the sudden flurry of action. The midwife will not take any chances now. If breathing is not clearly established she will hurry the baby off to a table where its lungs can be sucked out to clear any mucus which might have collected on the way out, and, if necessary to give oxygen through a face mask.

The baby's condition will be watched and, if breathing is not established quickly, it may be necessary for the baby to be taken into the special care unit for observation and help.

Records are now made of the baby's length, weight and head circumference as a baseline for future measurements which will give some guide to your baby's progress.

Identification bracelets will be checked with you and then fixed around the baby's wrists with your name and the baby's sex unless, of course, the birth takes place at home.

Third stage

Syntometrine is a drug which is usually administered during or just after delivery to expel the placenta. It is intended to stop excessive bleeding. This routine is not always necessary (see page 139).

Cutting the cord need not be done immediately. While the placenta is still attached, your baby is getting oxygen even if it isn't yet breathing, so it makes sense not to be too hasty in cutting it. However, if your baby doesn't start to breathe immediately, your midwife will lose no time cutting the cord and administering oxygen.

Delivering the placenta The midwife will put one hand on your tummy, to support your womb, and then pull gently on the cord with the other. If you have been given syntometrine this must be done within a few minutes before the cervix closes. If you have had no drugs, you will be asked to push the placenta out with your final contractions.

Tidying up

Stitches

'My legs are put in stirrups and I'm swathed in green cloths. I get ready to do my breathing but it doesn't hurt at all (was I just lucky). Mind you, I feel so high, he could have sawn my legs off and I wouldn't have batted an eyelid.'

If you have torn or had an episiotomy (cut) you will now be stitched up (see page 140). The stitching can take up to an hour, or sometimes more as there may be three layers to sew and the job should be done carefully. Some doctors are quite thoughtless and rough when stitching. They seem not to comprehend what a tiring and emotional experience you have just been through. Women have sometimes commented that they have been treated like 'a lump of meat'.

If your companion is with you during this stage it will be a comfort but you may well have to ask. Many hospitals routinely shoo them out. They reason that it is not the pleasantest view that your partner will ever have of you and, they think, perhaps better avoided.

A wash and change into a fresh gown will be a great pleasure now, followed by a cup of tea and, hopefully, a period alone with your companion and new baby.

COPING WITH PAIN

Now that drugs are available which are capable of relieving the pain of labour you may well ask why we should need to cope with pain at all?

The effective drugs which are available are not completely free from side effects. But even without these drawbacks, some women feel that a painfree labour is not as full an experience as an undrugged one. A woman in one survey on pain relief said, 'I had the birth removed from me.'

On the other hand if you are terribly nervous about labour you may well find that an epidural will give you confidence and make the birth a happier experience. If forceps delivery or Caesarean is considered likely, an epidural can give you freedom from pain and allow you to enjoy a delivery which might otherwise be very difficult.

In any case, you might like to read the sections on breathing and relaxation, as this will help whether or not you get the pain relief you want. Medical methods of pain relief are discussed in full on page 128.

Breathing, relaxation

There are a number of different techniques for managing a drug-free labour. It is always best to attend childbirth preparation classes, preferably with the companion who will be with you during labour. (If you are alone, you could ask a friend who has a child of her own to stay with you during labour. She will understand why you want company.) You cannot easily learn these techniques by reading, though just knowing about the progress of labour will be a big help.

Learning to breathe consciously will help you to relax; will ensure a continuous supply of oxygen through your blood to your baby; will give you something to hang on to which will help you to 'ride' the contractions and allow your womb to work as well as possible, unhindered by tense muscles.

Breathing patterns

There is no need to learn a set pattern though it helps to practise all kinds of breathing so that you can use them when necessary. Most women find that it works best to start off with deep breathing and then move up to high chest breathing and distraction at the peak of contractions. If you have a fast intense labour, you may want to use the distraction word (see below) most of the time.

1 *Relaxation techniques* described on page 85 will help you to keep your body from tensing up throughout labour. You may not manage during contractions but your companion can help you try to use the gaps in between to unlock any tensed-up muscles.
2 *Deep slow breathing*, concentrating on the out breath, will help you to relax in early labour.
3 *Chest breathing* again concentrating on breathing out, with a 'haaarrr' sound may feel more comfortable if deeper breaths start to press your diaphragm down uncomfortably

on your womb. Practise this by breathing with your hands on your ribs so that you can feel them moving in and out.

4 *High chest breathing* slowly and deliberately as though you were patting a candle flame ('huff, pause, huff, pause, huff') may help you at the top of the contraction. By concentrating on the out breath you prevent yourself from either holding your breath, and starving the baby of oxygen, or taking in too much and making yourself dizzy (hyperventilating).

5 *Hoo ha ha* is the sound to make at difficult moments. The definite rhythm as you breathe out (ignore the inbreaths, they will take care of themselves) provides a clear pattern to hang on to. Your partner will be able to help here by tapping out the rhythm on your arm, or clapping with you, to help you concentrate.

6 *Distraction* such as a song or chant to tap out, hum, sing or shout may help if the rhythm of the breathing doesn't seem to be enough to hold on to. You might want your partner to join in with you for encouragement, or, during the hardest part of labour, you may want to concentrate totally on your own body and find a duet distracting. Nicky remembered,

'I didn't want to take myself away from labour. When my contractions were very strong I chanted "open, open, open" to my cervix.'

7 *Over breathing* (hyperventilation) may make you feel dizzy and faint. You can feed a little more carbon dioxide back into your system to rebalance it by breathing into your cupped hands.

8 *Panting* Towards the end of the first stage of labour you may feel a tremendous urge to push. If the neck of your cervix is not fully open (about 10 cms dilated) the midwife will ask you to pant, or blow out, like a train. This is to stop you pushing too soon and bruising the cervix. You will find that the hoo ha ha breathing helps to control the pushing urge because it doesn't give you enough puff for a good push.

If you don't get to classes and all this sounds incomprehensible, the best way to cope is simply to concentrate on your own body and behave just the way you feel you need to. Change your position often, ask your partner to rub your back or apply pressure if it hurts, shout and yell if you need to, it doesn't matter in the least if you make a lot of noise. What you don't want to do is to panic, hold your breath and go stiff and rigid. Some women find that the most comfortable position is standing up and holding on to their companion as though dancing. This is a very good position to keep labour moving, and it will ensure that your labour remains a private affair.

DRUGS TO RELIEVE PAIN

In Britain 95 per cent of women giving birth will be given drugs for pain. In Holland, the figure is 5 per cent. Since there cannot be much difference between the women it seems likely that it is medical attitudes which differ. In Britain most midwives and doctors positively encourage women to opt for pain relief rather than giving them the support they need to manage without.

In fact there is only one form of drug which is capable of providing complete pain relief without knocking you out and that is an epidural. If you decide that this is what you want, then you must make sure it is available where you are booked, and that the hospital has been warned in advance that you want it. It is most easily set up quite early in labour but you may still be offered it later on if the pain gets worse than you feel able to cope with. However, once your labour is well advanced, you are more likely to be offered one of the other forms of pain relief described here.

Gas and air

A mixture of anaesthetic gas and oxygen (Entonox) is breathed in through a face mask. Anaesthetics called Penthrane and, more rarely, Trilene, may be given the same way. They make you feel a bit woozy and drunk.

It helps to try out the machine in the antenatal clinic or parentcraft class so that you get the hang of it before labour.

'I always panic if someone puts a hand over my nose, or I get ducked in a swimming pool. Just the thought of a gas mask made my stomach churn, but I found that with a little practice, I could hold the mask over my face and breathe quite normally.'

It is important to use the mask properly or it will either be totally ineffective or make you feel too dopey. The mixture takes about thirty seconds to work so you need to breathe it in before the peak of a contraction if the effect is to coincide with the pain.

Breathe in and out three or four times as soon as you feel a contraction starting and then put the mask down so that you can breathe your way over the crest of it. Don't let anyone else, even your lover, hold it over your face for you.

If the contractions are very sharp, your companion can help by putting the mask into your hand thirty seconds before the contraction is due.

If it takes a little while to get the gas and air working with the contractions, don't worry, just treat each new contraction as a new opportunity to get it right. Do not use the mask in the second stage. You will need to concentrate on pushing.

After effects   Entonox has no measurable after-effects on you or your baby. The other mixtures are a little stronger and you will probably absorb some but the effects won't last long.

Does it work?   Some women do find this a useful anaesthetic for a short time:

> 'When I was 6–7 centimetres dilated I was offered gas and air. I found it useful at this stage but, after fifteen minutes, I felt the urge to push and rejected the mask as it felt claustrophobic,'

said one mother.

Another commented,

> 'I couldn't get the gas and air thing going at all. I tried but it just didn't seem to be any help.'

Pethidine

This is given by injection in quantities between 50 and 200 mg. The effect takes about fifteen to twenty minutes to work. It should help you to relax, and a very low dose may be all you need to get a stubborn cervix to stretch the last little bit. You should always insist on an internal examination to check the progress of your labour before the drug is given. You may find that the knowledge that you've only got a little way to go will do you more good than any drug.

Additives   A variety of other drugs may be added to the pethi-

dine. Sparine is one which you should avoid. It has the unfortun-
ate side effect of making you forget the whole experience. Some
of the additives are intended to cut down nausea, others to increase the effect of the pethidine. None of them make it any
better for the baby.

Immediate effects   About 15 per cent of women find that the
pethidine makes them sick. It will also make you sleepy and, if
the dose is too high, it may even knock you out.

Some women enjoy the high 'floating' feeling it gives them.
Anne commented,

> *I'm usually very tense but I found I could easily relax between
> contractions and that I was calm and able to cope and so I
> was able to deal with the pain. Maybe it's because I'm a child
> of the sixties. I enjoy the feeling of being high and slightly out
> of control.'*

As a mood-continuous drug it will make you feel good if you are
already feeling good, but can make you feel bad if you were
feeling that way before it was given. The effects on you will wear
off in one and a half to two hours.

Disadvantages to the baby   Pethidine affects the baby's ability
to breathe properly. This side effect has been reduced by the use
of another drug, *narcan*, which is injected into you (just before)
or your baby (just after) birth and acts as an antidote. Nevertheless, a baby may be dopey at birth, slower to establish breathing,
slower to suck and generally sleepy until it has worked the stuff
out of its system.

You would have to be given the drug between six and eight
hours before delivery to ensure that the pethidine, and the breakdown products produced by your liver, had been completely
cleared from the baby's system. Clearly this early it is pretty
useless. If you have a little pethidine to relax the cervix in the
last hour or two before the birth, the drug will still be circulating
but, research indicates, the pethidine itself is easier for the baby's
immature system to cope with than the breakdown products from
your liver.

Either way it makes sense to ask for the lowest possible dose
to start with. The bigger your baby, the more easily he or she
will cope with drugs. Premature babies shouldn't be exposed to
them.

Does it work?   For those women who, like Anne, enjoy feeling high it can be calming and relaxing. However, most women agree that it doesn't actually help the pain.

> *'One minute I was lying on the bed in pain, a few minutes later I was floating near the ceiling – still in pain.'*

> *'Everyone around me seemed to think that the pethidine had done the trick. I knew it hadn't but I was too dopey to tell anyone. It made me panic.'*

Epidural anaesthesia
A local anaesthetic drug is injected directly into your spinal column where it numbs all feeling in your lower abdomen and legs. It has to be very precisely administered to go into the epidural space which lies between the bone of your spine and your spinal cord.

The procedure must be carried out by a skilled anaesthetist and takes from ten to twenty minutes. A local anaesthetic will be used and you have to lie curled up in a ball on your left side or sitting leaning forward. If you are having contractions, and feel one coming, say so and the anaesthetist will stop and start again when it's over.

A very fine tube (catheter) is inserted and stuck with tape up your back and over your shoulder. There is a plug in the end into which anaesthetic is injected. You can ask for a top-up dose as soon as you start to feel pain.

The procedure sounds unpleasant but, as Marianne wrote to the AIMS newsletter,

> *'I felt no pain when the catheter was inserted . . . a cold sensation but that was all. It was rather like having an injection at the dentist only less painful.'*

Immediate effects   The use of an epidural means that you will be having a medically managed labour. You will have to be monitored electronically and will have a drip set up to allow fluid to be fed through a needle into a vein in your arm in case your blood pressure drops – which is a possible side effect of an epidural. This means that you will be unable to move around or change your position very much.

The danger of a drop in blood pressure is increased if you lie on your back so you will have to stay on your side throughout the labour and will have a cuff on your arm so that your blood pressure can be easily checked.

The effect of lying down, combined with the effect of the anaesthetic, may slow things down a bit and that in turn may lead to the use of another drug, *syntocinon*, to speed up your labour. The second (pushing) stage will be strictly timed and, if the baby is not delivered in an hour, forceps may well be used.

Until recently, the forceps rate was extremely high with this form of pain relief, because midwives were timing the second stage from full dilatation rather than from the moment the head is seen. At Queen Charlotte's Maternity hospital in London the forceps rate was reduced when they started giving mothers a little longer in second stage.

You might get your companion to note down the time when the head is first seen. Then (provided the baby is not distressed) if forceps are suggested less than an hour later, you could ask for a little longer to try yourself.

Longer-term side effects Two out of every 100 women wind up with a crashing headache which keeps them flat on their backs for two days or more. Very occasionally some numbness in your legs persists for several weeks after the birth. These problems are less likely to occur with a highly experienced anaesthetist.

Effects on the baby If your blood pressure drops, this could reduce the supply of blood to the placenta and slow down the baby's heart rate.

Even though a local anaesthetic is used a little is transmitted to the baby through the bloodstream. Some forms of anaesthetic have been shown to affect the baby's ability to suck. If the use of an epidural means that the labour has been accelerated or forceps have been used the baby will have to contend with possible side effects from these procedures too.

Does it work? If it is properly inserted you should have a pain-free labour and a clear mind. Occasionally it doesn't work properly, or only works on one side of your body. If you had been expecting a pain-free labour and the anaesthetic was not effective you could find that very demoralising.

In some hospitals, the epidural is not topped up at the end of the first stage so that the mother can feel to push. This is probably an advantage as it means you are less likely to need forceps, but the sudden shock of late first-stage contractions may be absolutely overwhelming if there has been no slow build-up.

Nevertheless if it does work properly you will probably be delighted with it. Olivia Seligman wrote in *Honey* magazine about her labour,

'I really did lie back and enjoy it. I was able to watch the print-out of two monitors informing me that the contractions were getting more intense but also that my baby was coping with the strain. I felt deeply grateful that I was watching, rather than feeling, what looked like gargantuan peaks of pain appear on the print out.'

Pudendal block
This is a form of local anaesthetic which may be given if you need forceps to turn the baby or help it out and you have not had an epidural. The anaesthetic is injected into your vaginal wall about one finger-length up. The doctor will probably use a specially guarded needle to shield the baby's head and the anaesthetic should then numb the whole vaginal area and the perineum (the space between the vagina and anus).

Perineal infiltration
This is used to numb the perineal area between the vagina and anus when an episiotomy is performed. The injection is given straight into the perineum, and if the baby's head is already stretching the tissue you probably won't feel a thing. A low forceps 'lift out' may also be done with this form of local anaesthetic. If the doctor gives it a minute or two to work it should be quite effective.

Other methods of pain relief

Acupuncture is used in China as an anaesthetic. It involves putting very fine needles into certain points in your body (for labour it is usually the feet). Its disadvantage is that you cannot move around easily. There are varying reports as to how effective it is as a painkiller (see addresses on page 203).

Hypnosis is a very effective form of pain relief if you are susceptible to it (see page 203).

A pain relief machine is on trial at two British hospitals.

It uses a gentle electrical current to block your response to pain. As it is still very much in the experimental stage at present it is impossible to say whether it will be effective.

HOSPITAL PRACTICES

What we have described so far is the process of birth as it should be. Not every birth is straightforward. Sometimes that is because something has genuinely gone wrong and intervention is needed, urgently, to put it right. Jane had hoped for a straightforward GP unit delivery but it didn't go that way. Afterwards she wrote,

> *'It was very comforting to be amongst experts – foetal heart monitors put on, X-rays done. With the result they decided that a Caesarean was the only way to resolve things. It should have been discovered before.'*

Sadly hospital practices are often just routines which may get in the way of your enjoyment of the experience. If you know what is likely to be done to you and why, you, or your companion, can ask the right questions at the right time and ensure that you really need the things that are offered before accepting them.

Don't go into hospital assuming that it is the two of you together against technology. Taking an obviously informed interest is unlikely to put anyone's back up but you must be certain you are on strong ground before contradicting any suggestions put to you by medical staff. And (at risk of sounding patronising) do remember to be pleasant. This may be your first baby and the most important event in your life but to them it is a job, and you can help make it a pleasurable one.

Prepping

There are a number of procedures which are usually carried out in early labour.

Note-taking will always be the first step when you enter hospital. If you have made contact before going in your notes should be waiting for you in the labour ward. You will still be asked a number of questions, to ensure that you are definitely you, and about your labour.

Urine tests will be done now and whenever you pee, throughout labour, to ensure that you are not too low in energy, and to check for signs of infection.

Blood pressure is checked regularly during labour and after. If you are considered to be 'at risk' it will be taken more often.

An examination of your tummy and an internal examination will be done once you have changed from your outdoor clothes into a gown (yours or the hospital's). You will probably have your vulva and thighs washed down with an antiseptic solution first and the midwife will wear gloves (and possibly a gown) for the internal. She is checking the position of the baby and the dilatation (openness) of your cervix (neck of the womb).

Shaving will be necessary if you are having a Caesarean. Otherwise you can safely refuse. Shaving was originally introduced to cut down infection. Studies have now shown that it doesn't. In fact the tiny scratches left behind by the razor could encourage infection and the itching as the hair grows back is miserable. In progressive hospitals shaving won't even be suggested. In other places midwives may offer just to cut the hair back in the mistaken belief that it makes stitching easier. However it causes even more trouble because stubble grows into the stitches whereas long hair does not.

An enema, which is a tube of liquid or warm soapy water, is squirted up your back passage (anus). It is really only necessary if you are constipated in which case the waste matter in your bowel may obstruct the baby's head on the way out. Enemas have been discontinued as a routine in many hospitals because most women find them unpleasant and they are usually unnecessary as nature has already cleared your system.

If your waters have gone, and you are waiting for something to happen, an enema might help to start things off. It produces a fairly violent reaction which will send you racing to the toilet and may aggravate piles if you have them.

A warm bath is beautifully comfortable and relaxing. You may not want to get out. Unfortunately some hospitals have replaced bathing with a sponge down on a bed, successfully ridding their system of one of the only pleasant parts of preparations for labour.

Induction

> 'This is it, the excitement of knowing that I was actually going
> to have my baby overrode the 5.30 awakening. And no
> breakfast. Four impatient hours later I am wheeled out into
> the labour ward corridor. An hour and a half later, they
> remembered where they had put me and the induction process
> began.
>
> It took about half an hour to break the water (completely
> painless to my relief) and attach a monitor to the baby's head
> and me to a drip and all the relevant machinery. Labour
> started at 11.30.
>
> Emma slithered out at 4.27, what a marvellous
> experience. I can honestly say that I experienced no "pain" at
> any time apart from when I was trying not to push against a
> uterus that was pushing like fury, and so I was tensing up.'

Mandy's baby was induced after a false labour which started and
then didn't progress. It was followed a few days later by evidence
of raised blood pressure. She was told, after the birth, that the
induction had been necessary and that the placenta, which nour-
ishes the baby in the womb, had stopped functioning well. If you
turn back to page 99 you can read about the pros and cons of
induction.

If your labour is to be started artificially you will be asked
to come into hospital the evening before. In hospital, the following things are likely to happen.

1 Prostaglandin pessaries may be given before you go to sleep.
   These must be pushed right up into your vagina close to the
   cervix (neck of the womb). This should soften the cervix and
   may well trigger off labour with no further help. If it does
   not start labour it should at least make the syntocinon induction (see below) more successful and quicker. In some
   hospitals prostaglandin pessaries are used instead of syntocinon, which cuts out the need for a drip.
2 Your waters will be broken in the morning. Your feet are
   put in stirrups and then a vaginal examination will be done
   and the membrane holding your amniotic fluid (bag of
   waters) will be punctured with a little plastic hook or forceps.
   Doctor says this is painless though some women do find it

uncomfortable. It is known in medical jargon as an artificial rupture of the membranes (ARM).

3 A drip will be set up. This is a tube with a needle at the end which is put into a vein in your arm. It will be used to feed glucose and water (to give you energy) and syntocinon (synthetic oxytocin to start the contractions) into your blood stream.

You may have a machine called a Cardiff pump by your bed through which syntocinon is dripped automatically. This machine will increase the dose steadily. Sometimes the intensity of contractions is measured by a tube which is inserted into your womb and the dose will then be increased accordingly. A newer machine, an MM2, may be used to administer the drug. It switches to a very low dose when contractions are properly under way, increasing again if they get weaker.

You can always ask to have the dose turned down to the minimum once labour is established just to see if you can manage without it. The dose can be increased again if necessary but you will find the natural contractions easier to cope with than the syntocinon-induced ones.

Acceleration

Acceleration may be suggested if doctors feel that your labour has been going on too long with insufficient progress. The procedure is the same as for induction: synthetic oxytocin (syntocinon) will be dripped through a needle in your arm to stimulate contractions. The stronger contractions will cause similar side effects (see page 100).

In some hospitals acceleration has become routine. Your labour will be plotted on a graph (a *partogram*) showing the time, the amount of dilatation (stretching) of the neck of the womb, and the distance that the baby's head has travelled down. If your labour is slower than their 'norm' you will be given a drip to speed it up.

The idea is that a long labour tires both mother and baby and increases the risk of infection. The doctors feel that they are doing you a favour to speed things up. Of course they may well be right. If you have been in hard labour for hours and nothing is happening, you will probably be grateful for any assistance. However some doctors are a bit arbitrary about this decision:

> *'My waters broke at midday and, after an enema at 4 p.m., contractions were soon under way, coming every five minutes and lasting a minute. An hour later a young doctor strolled in. He didn't even speak to me, just looked at the chart at the end of the bed (which hadn't been changed for an hour) and said I should be accelerated. I was astonished and asked to be allowed to go it alone a little longer. I don't think he expected to be contradicted. Muttering darkly about infection risk he said he would give me two more hours to get going. By that time I was on my way to the delivery room. My baby was born at 9.45 without acceleration!'*

If, like Sarah quoted above, your labour has barely started, unless there is some specific medical reason there is no reason to start acceleration. Even in a long labour acceleration may be unwelcome. If your contractions are light, well spaced, and easy to cope with, and provided neither you nor your baby are tiring, there is really no need to accelerate. In fact, it may be worth staying at home a little longer just to avoid the use of drugs to hurry things along.

Helping yourself
If your labour has slowed down, you may find that getting up and walking around, standing, or squatting or a hot bath, will get things going again. As we mentioned earlier, breast stimulation releases natural oxytocin. Otherwise you could ask for a prostaglandin pessary instead of a drip as this may have the desired effect in a gentler way.

Other routines

An electronic monitor is used routinely in some hospitals. It is essential if you are having an epidural and is usually used for an induced or accelerated labour.

You will be monitored both to trace your contractions – through a belt around your tummy or a *catheter* in your womb – and to trace your baby's heartbeat – through a second external belt or an internal scalp electrode which is attached to the baby's head. Doctors consider the scalp electrode to be more accurate though we cannot be certain how the baby feels about it. It does often leave a sore and, occasionally, a bald patch. If your waters haven't already broken they will be pierced in order to attach the monitor. For a description of how to interpret monitors look on page 97.

A major drawback with monitoring is that you cannot move around easily (unless you are lucky enough to be in a hospital which has remote control *telemetry* equipment). If you cannot move easily your labour may well last longer and feel more painful. Ironically this could actually lead to the baby tiring which is just what the monitor is there to record.

If there is no obvious reason why you should be monitored, and you want the freedom to move around during labour, you could ask the midwives if they would mind monitoring you with a portable sonic aid or pinnard.

A drip may be required to feed energy directly into your bloodstream if a urine sample shows that you have been too long without food. A solution of dextrose and water will be fed through a needle into a vein in your arm.

An injection of Syntometrine is routinely given to you just as the baby is being delivered. This drug makes your womb contract to deliver the placenta. The contractions will close off the blood vessels which have linked you with the baby. Your body's natural oxytocin should perform the task quite adequately but if for some reason it doesn't you are in danger of a *postpartum haemorrhage* (PPH) which used to be a major cause of maternal death.

Although the routine use of Syntometrine appears to have cut the risk of PPH it does have side effects: your blood pressure may suddenly rise (it should be used with caution if you already have high blood pressure); it may make you vomit; and it sometimes causes the neck of the womb to close before the placenta has been delivered in which case it would have to be removed under a general anaesthetic. One study also showed that milk production was delayed by the Ergometrine component of Syntometrine so, in some hospitals, pure Syntocinon is used instead.

Those women most at risk of PPH will have had: many pregnancies; a twin pregnancy; ante-partum haemorrhage; or a history of PPH. If you are not in a risk category you could ask the midwife not to use syntometrine unless you actually start to bleed. If it is injected straight into a vein it works in forty-five seconds.

Episiotomy

This is the medical name for the cut which may be made in the perineum to help the baby out. Just thinking about it may make you squirm but you really shouldn't feel it at all. If the cut is made, as it should be, when the baby's head is stretching the perineum (see picture) it should feel numb. If there is time you may be given a local anaesthetic injection two minutes before it is done to make double sure. After the birth you should be given a second local anaesthetic injection, which must be given time to take effect, before the cut is stitched. If the stitching hurts, say so, and ask the doctor to stop and wait until the anaesthetic has taken effect.

Episiotomy should be carried out for a reason, not just for medical convenience or routine.

Reasons for episiotomy are: for a forceps delivery; to help out a baby who is in difficulty; to speed delivery of a premature baby (though this is also being questioned now); in most cases for breech births; and when a severe tear looks likely.

A number of other reasons may be given for the routine use of episiotomy but they are not backed up by any convincing research. One suggestion is that a perineum which is allowed to stretch may, in later years, cause the ligaments supporting the womb to sag (a prolapse). There is no evidence that this is so.

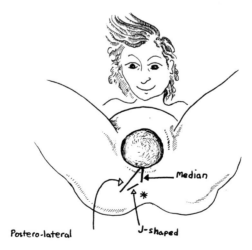

Episiotomy incisions

Another really crazy reason is that a stitched perineum will be tighter and therefore sex will be better. Evidence from women indicates that a stitched vagina makes sexual intercourse painful for some weeks and occasionally for considerably longer. The idea of stitching a woman into shape suitable for male gratification is a revolting practice and should be universally condemned.

Evidence is now overwhelming that a small tear heals more quickly causing less discomfort than a cut. Scissors need only be used where there is a clear need, for the baby's sake, or where a deep (third-degree) tear looks likely.

Helping yourself

You can help to make an episiotomy unnecessary by adopting a good position for delivery (see page 120) and practising pelvic floor exercises during pregnancy. When you can feel your baby's head stretching the skin of your perineum (see page 121) you may then be able, consciously, to relax your pelvic floor muscles and so help the baby out rather than holding her in.

Mention to your midwife that with her help you would like to avoid an episiotomy if at all possible.

'I heard the midwife say that she would need to cut. I pulled myself together and said: "I know I will thank you if you don't." That seemed to provide the encouragement she needed to manage his delivery without using scissors. I did tear slightly but the tear healed far quicker and less painfully than the cuts some of my friends suffered.'

Forceps

These are long instruments a bit like two spoons which may be used if for any reason it is considered wise to get the baby out faster than you can manage yourself. They may also be used to turn a baby from a difficult position to one which is easier for delivery, and to protect the head of a tiny premature baby.

In some hospitals, forceps are used automatically if the second (pushing) stage is delayed longer than an hour for a first baby or half an hour for other babies.

While forceps are undoubtedly life-saving in some circumstances there may not be any need to use them for a delayed second stage provided your baby is still in good shape. Your companion could ask why they are considered necessary if there does not seem to be any urgency (but don't expect a patient explanation at this stage).

Your legs will be put up in stirrups. A local anaesthetic will be used if you have not already had an epidural. Then a fairly large cut (episiotomy) must be made to allow the doctor to slide in the forceps, a blade at a time. The forceps are curved and they lock in position so that they cup the baby's head rather than grasping it. The baby can then be pulled out.

Barbara knew that her baby needed to be delivered quickly because she could hear his heartbeat on the monitor beginning to get erratic.

'The doctor gave me a local anaesthetic injection in my perineum [the area between your vagina and anus]. I knew he would have to do a cut and then slide in the blades but I really couldn't feel which was which. It didn't hurt at all.'

The forceps used were Wrigleys which are only used to lift out a baby who has nearly made it unaided. If longer forceps are used to pull a baby down, a pudendal block may be given (see page 133).

Vacuum extraction (ventouse) is sometimes used instead of forceps, both for turning and delivering the baby. A suction cap is placed on the baby's head and then suction applied by a machine. You can usefully push at the same time to help the baby out. Its advantage over forceps is that it can be used before your cervix is fully dilated, whereas forceps cannot.

Caesarean section

This may be planned in advance for one of the reasons mentioned on page 101, or done in an emergency because: forceps are unsuccessful; your pelvis proves to be too small; the cord prolapses (comes out ahead of the baby); the cervix fails to open; or the baby shows signs of severe distress.

The usual signs that your baby is distressed are: a heart monitor reading showing 'type two dips' (see page 97); a blood sample showing that the baby is not getting enough oxygen; or a slowing heart rate discovered through a sonic aid. Greenish black staining in your waters (meconium) shows that your baby has had a bowel movement and that may also be an initial indicator of distress which would be checked.

While the operating theatre is prepared, your pubic hair will be shaved and a catheter inserted to drain off any urine which collects during the operation. A glucose drip will then be attached to your arm. All this preparation will be done before you are anaesthetised (in the case of a general anaesthetic) to ensure that you are given the lightest possible dose of drugs so that your baby doesn't absorb much.

If it is an emergency Caesarean, and you have not already had an epidural anaesthetic, you will probably be given a general. Vivienne had a planned Caesarean this way:

'I had to inhale oxygen for the baby, then I felt something very cold going through the needle into the back of my hand. I started to have the most incredible dream. I was going through the alphabet and as I got to Z the pain got more intense. I was aware of voices coming soft and loud saying "we've got a beautiful boy, we've got our Gareth". When I finally gathered my senses I remember asking the time. It was 11.30 and the baby was born at 10 a.m. I can remember Ivor saying "do your breathing exercises" and that the sun was shining and what a beautiful day for our baby to be born.'

If you have already had an epidural, or if you planned your Caesarean in advance you may prefer to have the operation under epidural anaesthesia which leaves you awake and clear-headed during the procedure and afterwards. It uses far fewer anaesthetic drugs than you would need for a general. That means that your baby will suffer less from side effects (see page 101 for Linda's experience).

You will be aware of what goes on but will feel no pain. As one woman put it, 'it felt as if they were rummaging around inside me.'

You won't actually see the operation because a screen will be put up. You may feel the cut as if a pencil were being drawn across your tummy. In most cases a small, horizontal 'bikini' incision will be made.

Then you will hear the glugging noise of a suction instrument which draws off the water the baby has been floating in, and your baby will be lifted out. If all is well she, or he, may be wrapped and handed to you to hold while you are being stitched up.

If you have had a Caesarean under general anaesthetic you will want to know that your baby is being loved while you are sleeping. Your companion can take a very positive part in the birth by caring for the baby in these first few minutes of life. Here is one father's account of an emergency Caesarean:

' "Would you like to take him into the nursery or stay with your wife?" I look across at her. She is asleep. I look at the baby. His arms are locked in the stiff clothing and the light is burning his eyes. "With him" I say.

I sit with my son in my arms. We are both crying. The nurse comes, turning on a bright light. "Now let's clean it up," she says. "I expect you'll think me a bit soft," I say quietly, "but I want to bath him." "You fathers! Well, if you insist." I take him from the cloth. His tiny body is slippery. I support him in my arms and lower him into the water slowly.'

Once the effects of a general anaesthetic have worn off you will feel the pain that anyone would experience just after an operation which has cut through a layer of muscles. Painkillers will be offered to relieve the discomfort but you will probably want to be awake as much as possible to get to know your baby. You may also feel sick and muzzy-headed for a day or two.

With an epidural you should not have these problems. It will be left in for a few hours after the birth so you should not have so much need of painkillers for post-operative pain. You will not have that muzzy-headed feeling either.

Whichever method of anaesthetic is used, it is important to get moving as soon as possible to stir your blood circulation and aid recovery. A chair next to the bed will help you get in and out. Try using the breathing exercises described on page 126 to ease the pain while you do so.

After a general anaesthetic you will have a sore throat from the tubes put into your stomach, and your lungs will be full of fluid which may be quite painful to cough up. This is how Vivienne managed:

'Draw up knees, cup hands over tummy, tighten buttocks, and drop back on to the bed. It takes a little while but it works.'

Breastfeeding may seem difficult too, partly because your milk may take a little longer to come:

'I lay on my side and the nurse rested him on a pillow under

my arm at first. After the first couple of days I asked if I could
feed him sitting on a chair with a pillow on my tum. It was
much more comfortable.'

You can expect a hospital stay of about ten days. No bathing for
the first three or four days.

Special care

If your baby seems unwell at birth, if she is premature, suffering
from infection or from physical handicap, she may be taken into
special care. Even if there is very little wrong, it may be traumatic to be parted from her so soon. Fiona felt that those first
hours after the birth were when she most needed to have her
companion with her:

'I hadn't slept for forty-eight hours and I was all alone. The
paediatrician came into the ward to take my baby to special
care for an antibiotic drip. I said, "No way, I want my baby
with me." I insisted on going too and they wheeled me down
with the baby on my knee. A nurse tried to take her away but
I wouldn't let her. Then, when they put a needle into her arm,
I started to cry. They just wanted to get on with it. In the end
I agreed to go.'

Medical staff are beginning to realise how very important it is
for a mother and baby to spend their first days together. If your
baby is tiny, and wired up to tubes attached to machines, you
may feel very nervous. Those tubes are there to help your baby
over the first hurdles of breathing and eating, until she can
manage adequately on her own. Underneath she is still a baby,
your baby, and she needs your close attention and love as much
as the food and oxygen.

Ask the staff exactly why she is there and how long she is
likely to stay. Try, if you can, to feed her yourself. If she cannot
suck, ask if you can use an electric pump to express your milk
for her. If this isn't possible for some reason, see if the hospital
has a milk bank. A sick baby has a particular need for the
protective properties of breast milk.

If the baby dies

It is hard to imagine a more intense pain than the loss of a baby who has never lived. It is the harder to bear because there is no one to share it with. Only you, who carried the baby, and your partner, who shared the birth, will ever have known her.

Most parents who have lived through this experience feel that it is better to see the child you have borne. It is easier to heal the loss of a baby you can picture than to come to terms with the images that your imagination will put in her place.

If she hangs on to life in special care, the waiting will be a terrible strain, but you will be able to look back with the knowledge that you had the opportunity to love your baby for as long as she lived.

Grief shared is easier to cope with. Organisations which provide counselling and support are listed on page 203.

Chapter 6

A NEW LIFE

HOW DO YOU FEEL?

'They wheeled me down to the ward and I could see a beautiful full moon and I could hear people singing carols and I felt so good – I just wanted to go outside and roll in the grass. I hardly slept all night. I felt so high I could have floated round the ward. It was lovely and I've felt lovely ever since.'

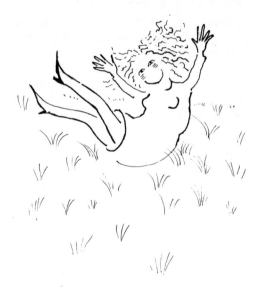

That feeling of exhilaration is wonderful but it isn't quite so immediate for everyone:

'John went home to sleep and I felt bereft. The experience had been so close and intense and now I was all alone – not

counting the twenty other women in the ward. That first night I hardly slept. At 6 a.m. my curtains were flung back and there he was, open-mouthed and yelling. I felt stupid and incompetent and alone. When the morning rituals of breakfast and bathing were out of the way I phoned home but nothing came out of me except sobs. Oddly enough, within two hours I had zoomed up into the stratosphere and stayed there for the next fortnight.'

You may well enjoy the bustle of the ward and the company of other new mothers. On the other hand, conflicting advice, or even a badly timed comment from a member of staff or neighbour can knock you sideways. A young mother, quoted in Valerie Welburn's book, *Post Natal Depression* put the feeling well:

'I think you are very vulnerable, ever so vulnerable. It's a bit of a tightrope, isn't it? You've got to get across. I think you know you are going to get there, but if the wrong person is there at the wrong time it can affect you.'

If you do feel unhappy in hospital, and long to be at home with people you love, you can always discharge yourself, provided there are no medical reasons for keeping you in and you will have plenty of help at home. You are better off happy at home than sad in hospital. Just ask for a paediatrician to check your baby over, and if she is well, tell the ward sister you are leaving. The hospital will ensure that you are visited daily, at home, by a district midwife.

Partners' feelings

Partners' feelings can very easily be overlooked now, but they too have been through a very emotional experience. Elation may be mixed with anxiety, and loneliness:

John said,

'I was pretty relieved to get home to bed. I was very, very tired, but I soon found myself in an uncomfortable limbo. Still working, trying to get the house finished, and visiting the hospital twice a day. I was impatient to get them home, but fearful that once they got here, my life would have totally changed.'

If your partner is to take a real share in the care and upbringing of this baby then the first hours, and days, after the birth are important.

Mothers who are separated from their babies in the first days may have more difficulty 'bonding' with them. How much more difficult must it be for someone who does not have the help of that special closeness which comes with feeding? Life with a new baby can be pretty gruelling. It is the love and the fierce protective feeling developed in these first days which will carry you through the next few months. Your partner needs a chance to share that feeling. If you are in hospital, that closeness is going to be cut down:

'We had always intended to share her care but, by the time I got home from hospital, I had already developed a certain expertise. He felt clumsy and inadequate. When Joanna started to cry he felt powerless to comfort her. She only calmed down when I fed her and he couldn't do that. I could feel him drawing away, getting angry and impatient when she cried, and there seemed to be nothing we could do about it. I can't help thinking that if he had had a role to play from the start, his love for her would have overcome his feeling of helplessness.'

It may help to set aside one visiting time, or a particular time of day, when you can be alone together to make sure that your partner learns what you are learning and has as much contact with the baby as possible. Even a sleeping baby can be cuddled.

This sharing is not nearly as easy as it sounds. It needs working at. Jane and Bob came home together hours after the birth of their first child:

'I was very uncomfortable what with my stitches and, after a couple of days, painful breasts too. The midwife taught Bob how to bath and change the baby. He took over all of that leaving me to provide food. I felt that the baby had nothing to do with me. All I was good for was providing milk. It took a long time for me to get the confidence even to put on a nappy competently.'

There are going to be times when establishing a balance seems impossible. You don't want to let go, your partner doesn't do enough. In time you will all get to know each other and a pattern will emerge.

YOUR BODY AFTER THE BIRTH

Vaginal bleeding After the first four days, the blood should get browner. If it stays bright red, mention it to your midwife. As the bleeding decreases you may get a heavy, thick, white discharge which is occasionally blood-stained. It can last for up to six weeks. You may notice a sudden gush of blood each time the baby suckles to start with, and sometimes after about ten days.

Heavy bleeding, or an offensive smell, should be reported. It may be evidence of a retained piece of placenta, or of infection. If you find any blood clots on your pads, keep the pad in a bag to show the midwife. She needs to ensure that it is just blood and not a piece of placenta.

Pads should be provided by the hospital (though government expenditure cuts are stopping this practice in some hospitals). You should use these sterile pads for the first two days. After that you may prefer to provide your own. Extra long maternity pads are more comfortable because they don't rub your stitches.

After pains are more common after second and subsequent babies. Try using the breathing technique described for labour. If the pain is troubling you, ask for a mild pain killer.

Constipation may worry you, especially if you have stitches. Don't even expect a bowel movement for two to three days. Your system was completely cleared during labour. Eat a particularly high fibre diet (did you take a bag of bran into hospital?) and drink plenty of fluids now so that, when you do go, it won't hurt. The tenderness of your perineum may be off-putting but putting it off will make things worse. A midwife will suggest a mild laxative if nothing has happened by the third day. If you are not prone to constipation there is no reason why it should start now but, at a tender moment like this, you may be grateful for some extra help!

Avoid infection by washing frequently. If there is a handy shower available, wash yourself between the legs after each bowel movement. Change your pad frequently.

Piles can be even more painful than stitches. Your midwife will give you pessaries and cream to soothe and shrink them (see page 57 for tips).

Pee as soon as you can after the birth. You should pee a great deal in the first hours and days. If you don't or have trouble doing so, or find that you haven't done so for many hours after the birth, you should mention it. Very occasionally, the tube can get bruised during labour and the swelling may temporarily block it, in which case the midwife will have to empty your bladder for you using a catheter.

Wind is also quite common. It will soon ease.

Aftercare of stitches Whether you have had a cut or a tear, your stitches will be uncomfortable for a while. It helps to take a child's rubber ring into hospital to sit on. This will take the pressure off the tender area when you sit down.

Bathing several times a day is very soothing. If peeing stings, try pouring warm water over the stitches at the same time. An old detergent bottle filled with water is a convenient aid.

Dry yourself carefully, preferably with a hairdryer. Dry stitches heal more quickly.

Comfrey ointment can be applied to the sore areas (you can get it from health food shops and some chemists).

Exercise your pelvic floor muscles (see page 8) as soon as you can. It will aid healing and start toning them up again.

In the days after the birth, as the stitches shrink you may feel pain, but after a week they should heal rapidly. However, you may feel tenderness for considerably longer than this. Gentle exploration with your fingers will keep you informed of the condition of your perineum. Don't do anything to hurt it. (See page 178 on sex.)

Heat treatment: if you have a reading lamp by your bed, draw the curtains and shine the light on your perineum.

Exercise will be demonstrated by a physiotherapist or midwife (ask if they don't mention it) to aid blood circulation and healing and return your muscles to their pre-pregnant state. It helps to get out of bed and walk around as soon as possible too.

Your breasts will start to swell on about the third day as your milk comes in. This can be quite painful. You may be alarmed at the size of them. If you are breastfeeding, the fullness and hardness will gradually decrease the more often your baby suckles, and establishes a balance between her needs and your supply. Otherwise a tight-fitting bra will suppress lactation but you will have large, sore, hard breasts for several days.

Weepiness is a very common accompaniment to swelling breasts. The initial excitement of the birth is over, you may feel uncomfortable and your hormone supply is readjusting. In fact, weepiness doesn't necessarily mean that you actually feel sad.

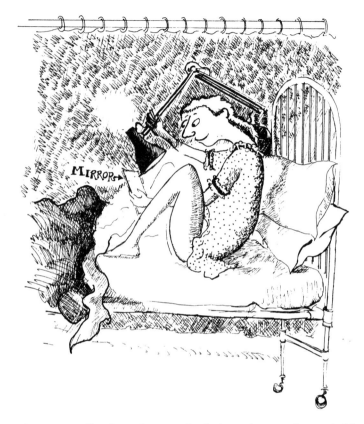

If you have a reading lamp by your bed, draw the curtains and shine the light on your perineum

'In those early days I cried about everything but it was mostly from happiness. I did feel an idiot when people said: "What a lovely baby" and I felt myself starting to cry. I just had to explain to people not to worry about the water works.'

If you have other worries at this time, this emotional upheaval can make you feel very low. Some hospital staff may dismiss your feelings as unimportant because it is 'just hormones'. Try to shut your ears to such thoughtlessness. You have just been through a shattering experience, you are tired and quite weak. No wonder you feel delicate. What you need now is someone to 'mother' you.

Routine aftercare
For the first ten days a midwife is obliged to see you daily, whether you are in hospital or at home.

Your temperature and pulse will be checked morning and evening for the first three days and every day for the next seven.

Your blood pressure is checked after delivery and on the tenth day.

Your tummy will be felt (palpated) to ensure that your uterus is shrinking and your bladder is functioning properly. The midwife may measure your tummy with a ruler to check the rate of its decrease in size (involution).

Your perineum will be inspected to see that the stitches are healing and to check for any bruising or swelling which might need treatment. Your pad will be checked and the colour and consistency of the blood noted.

A blood test will be taken after a couple of days to check for any sign of anaemia. If you have been taking iron during pregnancy, continue to take it for the first six weeks after the birth.

HOW DO YOU FEEL ABOUT YOUR BABY?

'We looked at each other. Any thoughts of previous preference were swept away. Boy, girl, fair, dark, such distinctions were meaningless. He was quite definitely just himself gazing up solemnly. His body was softer than anything I could imagine. He sucked vigorously, burped, sighed and went to sleep.'

If you don't feel immediately overwhelmed with love and tenderness for your baby, don't be alarmed. According to one study, about 40 per cent of first-time mothers are less than enchanted with their babies for the first two or three days.

Women whose labours had not been straightforward, who had large doses of pethidine, or who found the pain of labour worse than they expected, were most likely to feel a bit detached to start with but, fortunately, familiarity in this case seems to breed love. By the end of the first week almost all the mothers questioned felt pretty soppy about their babies. For some it took longer.

Routine aftercare of the baby

The cord will be examined each day to ensure that it is clean and uninfected. You will be shown how to wipe it with surgical spirit or water and dust it with cord powder to keep it clean and dry. It should drop off on or before the tenth day.

Weight will be checked every three days for the first ten days. Babies usually lose about 100 to 200 grams in the first three days (which will be put back on some time over the next couple of weeks), and then gain weight fairly steadily. Don't worry about graphs and norms. If your baby is gaining rather than losing and seems bright-eyed, alert and a good colour, with vigorous movement, you needn't worry about weight.

Hips will be checked before you leave hospital, or within ten days, by your doctor or a paediatrician. A few babies are born with dislocated hips. Often it is only necessary to put a double nappy on to coax the hips back. Occasionally splints may be necessary.

Reflexes are checked within forty-eight hours. A baby who is born at forty weeks will usually respond in a certain way to a stimulus: if you hold the baby horizontally and allow her head to drop back slightly, she will throw out her arms (the Moro reflex). If you put a finger in her palm, she will grasp it and if you pull her up to a sitting position she will pull back against you. If the baby is held upright with her feet on a hard surface, she will make stepping movements with her legs. Finally, if you touch her cheek, she will turn towards the touch and open her mouth (the rooting reflex). Some of these reflexes will fade after the first few days until your baby is bigger and strong enough to make use of them.

Rashes will be noted. A 'milk rash' may appear and then disappear in the first two weeks.

Blood spots may be seen in a girl baby's nappy, in the first few days. This is because your hormones have been suddenly withdrawn from her system. Her womb responds to hormones just as yours does.

Breasts of both boy and girl babies may swell slightly in the first three days. This is also a response to hormones. Just leave them alone and the swelling will subside.

A Guthrie test will be done on a blood sample from the baby's heel, a check for a rare disorder called phenylketonuria.

Jaundice is a very common condition in the first few days.

The baby's skin goes yellowish (a black baby's jaundice is most noticeable in the whites of the eyes). It happens because the liver is having difficulty getting rid of extra red blood cells which it no longer needs now that the baby is breathing. The best treatment is exposure to sunshine. You may be asked to give the baby extra water. If you are breastfeeding just feed more frequently. In any case a mild case will clear in a few days.

Jaundice which starts before the second day, or seems severe, will need treatment. A blood test will be taken from the heel to check on the reason for, and severity of the jaundice. The baby may have to spend time in special care, under a light. A mask will be put over her eyes to protect them. You can just take it off when you feed her.

Circumcision is never necessary at this stage for medical reasons. The foreskin on the penis cannot be pulled back because it has not yet separated from the bit underneath. It is therefore impossible to say whether the child will have future problems with it. You should not try pulling a baby's foreskin back because you might cause damage.

'Our baby is different'

> *'The main point which I feel needs shouting about is that she is a baby; not a Down's baby or a mongol, but a baby with her own individual personality and character.'*

All they had known before her birth was that Chloe would be light for dates. She was delivered by Caesarean and turned out to weigh less than five pounds with a heart defect and Down's syndrome (these things often go together). Zelda won't ever forget the mixture of shock and concern for her baby:

> *'I was told by this big-nosed man in a white coat that there were two things wrong with her and that her life was in danger. He would say nothing more until my husband was there. My only feeling then was for Chloe. My mind flashed back to an article I had read about a baby with Down's syndrome being allowed to die. God, was I scared. I just shouted at him, "Don't just stand there, do something, save her."*
>
> *I wanted to see her and she was brought to me, with her*

*eyes closed and swaddled like a Victorian doll. She was tiny,
and fragile and beautiful.'*

For Zelda, the twelve days in hospital with Chloe's incubator in
her room were 'horrible', but she feels:

*'Chloe and I had been through something so awful together
that it had brought us closer. At seven months she is now a
beautiful child. Still tiny, but very alert and wide-eyed, and
can already sit up. She has already achieved so much more
than they said she would and she gives me a great deal of joy.'*

There is not the space in this book to go very deeply into the
special problems that you will face if your baby is born with a
handicap. You will inevitably feel a mixture of anger, grief and
disappointment and possibly even guilt.

All these feelings are quite understandable. Our society is
not very loving towards people who are different and you would
be unusual if you did not fear for your child's future.

You will need a great deal of extra help in, first of all, clearly
identifying the problems (see page 182), researching the possibility of treatment and then finding ways of helping your child
to live to the limit of his or her own potential.

You may fear for your own future too, but even if the handicap is serious, it need not be the end of your life as an
individual.

Julia's son is now 14 months old. He was born with a severe
mental handicap.

*'He looked perfectly normal at birth but his development was
extremely slow. We didn't know for definite what was wrong
until he was a year old. I was totally disoriented. It took away
all our expectations. David was absolutely shattered and it
was years before we could really talk about it. It was the
support of friends which made the difference. Our best friends
were even able to take him away for weekends to give us a few
breaks.*

*I have never stopped my own work and my own life. To
start with I just did any part-time work I could to earn
enough money for an au pair. He started a day nursery at
eighteen months and then went on to a special school. We
built his exercises into our daily routine, around meals, and
in the evenings, and we took him with us wherever we went.*

*We simply carried on just as we would have done if he had
been a normal child.*

*He has had to be taught everything: sitting, standing,
walking. Now he can do quite a lot for himself. I'm terribly
proud of his achievements because I know how hard he works
to do the tiniest things. When we had him, friends told us
that, in many other cultures, people who have children like
ours are considered blessed – chosen. We have been picked
because we have special strength. It helps to think of it like
that. I know he has given me strength.'*

FEEDING IN THE FIRST SIX MONTHS

Breast and bottle-feeding are often discussed as though there
was little to choose between them but convenience. In fact, they
are quite different. Dried, powdered, cow's milk (formula) is a
substitute for the real thing. It is a good substitute, and just as
many people are untroubled by the difference between acrylic
and wool, your baby may manage pretty well on bottle milk.
However, there are several major differences between these two
foods:

1 Cow's milk has a different proportion of the different food-
   stuffs in it. It is not digested so easily and as a result,
   bottle-fed babies tend to go longer between feeds and produce
   more in their nappies.
2 The 'foreign protein' in cow's milk can trigger off an allergy
   to dairy products in a sensitive baby. If you have allergies
   in your family (eczema, asthma or hay fever) you would be
   wise to avoid any cow's milk products for the first six months;
   even one bottle may trigger off an allergy.
3 Antibodies, produced by your body to fight against disease,
   are passed on through your milk, particularly in the colostrum, which is waiting in your breasts when your baby is
   born. This gives a breastfed baby some protection against
   disease in the early months when it has no protective antibodies of its own. These antibodies do not occur in treated
   cow's milk. So bottle-fed babies are more vulnerable to
   infection.
4 Hygiene is not a problem with breastfed babies because the
   milk is never exposed to bacteria. Scrupulous hygiene is
   necessary with bottles to avoid introducing bacteria.

These are the differences we know about, there may be other differences which we don't yet appreciate. Just as you will be healthier if you eat food which is as close as possible to its natural state, your baby will also do better on the milk which is tailored to it than an 'off the peg' substitute.

Why don't we all breastfeed?

Shyness about feeding in public or even in front of family and friends may put you off. It is a great pity that we have such a distorted view of women's bodies in Western society. Everywhere we look we are bombarded with images of the naked female form put there for the amusement of passing men. Yet if we want to use our breasts for a useful purpose, we fear that people will be shocked.

In fact, you may well find that you are strangely brazen once you actually do start feeding your baby.

'I had expected to feel really shy about feeding him in public, but once I had worked out a way of doing it fairly discreetly, I did it everywhere. People looked faintly surprised at first but as long as I wasn't bothered, they stopped noticing.'

It would be a pity to let embarrassment about feeding stop you from going out with your baby. It is so much more convenient than bottles.

'He came everywhere with me in those early weeks. A couple of spare nappies in my handbag and I was equipped. There was never any rush to get home. He just snuggled up in the sling to sleep, and whenever he started nudging at me for a drink I'd draw my shawl around both of us and let him suck.'

If you wear clothes that can be pulled up from the waist, rather than buttoning down the front, you will be able to feed discreetly.

Of course, there are other reasons why women don't start breastfeeding, or stop very soon. You can read about them in the section on feeding problems on page 162. If you begin with breastfeeding even if you cannot continue you will have given your baby the best possible start.

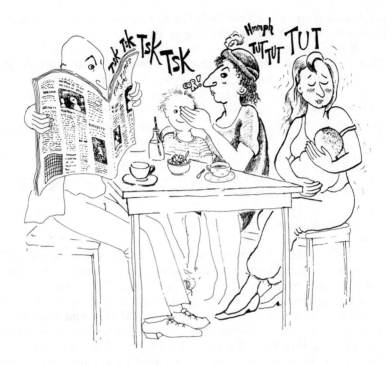

How breastfeeding works

The baby is one side of a system. Suckling sends messages to your breast to produce more milk. The more the baby suckles, the larger the quantity of the milk you produce. If your baby feeds frequently, the supply and demand will keep pace. If feeds are spaced there may be a bit of a time lag.

If you give your baby extra milk from a bottle she won't demand extra from you. What she doesn't ask for, you won't supply and your milk supply will start to dwindle. If you feel unhappy about your milk supply see page 162.

Your body is the other side of the system. There is always a little milk in the milk glands behind your nipples, but most of it is locked in until you let it out. This is called your *let down reflex*. Presumably it is nature's way of ensuring that you don't drip all the time. To stop leaking, when it does occur, press the nipple hard with the heel of the hand.

You may feel your let down reflex working as a strange

tingling feeling, a bit like the build-up to a sneeze. Some women let down without feeling anything at all.

If you are relaxed, the reflex will start to work as soon as your baby starts to suckle. The message may take a couple of minutes to get through at first and your baby may get quite cross waiting for something to happen. Once you have started to establish a rhythm you may find the tingling starts as soon as you hear a baby (any baby!) cry and then the milk is ready waiting in your breasts at the start of a feed.

'If I was out without him I would have to try not to think about him around his feed time because I would start to leak.'

Establishing breastfeeding in hospital

In some hospitals dextrose and water are given routinely to all newborn babies. This is not necessary if your baby is healthy, although the extra energy boost may be needed, for example, for very small premature, or chilled babies. Ask to speak to the paediatrician about it before it is given. If you find that it is necessary for your particular baby, ask if it would be all right to try breastfeeding first. If a baby gets her first few drinks mainly from a bottle it can confuse her feeding programme and may make breastfeeding harder to establish.

Hospitals may also insist that your baby stay in the nursery for the first two nights. This is meant to give you a rest. If you want your baby with you, say so; if you are happy for the break but keen to breastfeed, put a note on the cot stating that your baby should not be given formula but must be brought to you for feeding if she cries. A single bottle of milk can trigger an allergy.

Sleeping pills may be offered in the first night or two. This is partly because you may be too 'high' to sleep and partly an acknowledgment of how noisy and disturbing a hospital ward can be. However, drug-induced sleep is not as restful as even two hours of normal sleep, after breastfeeding. Your baby will also be absorbing the drug and just one dose can take three days to clear from the system. This may make her sleepy and lethargic about feeding.

How to feed your baby

Immediately after birth, babies who are not heavily drugged are very alert. The suckling instinct is strong and, if your baby finds out what to do with it, you will have few problems establishing feeding. Lift your baby to your breast and see what happens. If no interest is shown, try again in a little while.

If you don't have the opportunity or your baby doesn't have the inclination, then try as soon as you can. Here is what to do.

Sit comfortably with your back supported, or (specially if you have had a Caesarean) lie with the baby beside you. If you are not in a comfortable position, you will probably try to hurry things and that won't be a very good start. Hold your baby in the crook of your arm. If it seems more comfortable, lay her on a cushion on your lap.

Rooting is the curious birdlike seeking for your breast which you should notice if you just hold your baby with her face against your breast. The baby will turn instinctively *towards* anything which touches her cheek. So if you try to push her towards your breast you may well find that she moves her mouth in the wrong direction. If you stroke the cheek nearest your nipple she should turn towards it.

Latching on If your baby is to get milk, she must squeeze the milk ducts just behind the nipple with her gums. In order to get the pressure in the right place, your nipple must be right back in her mouth. Some books will say that you must get the whole of the dark area (*areola*) in her mouth. This is just a guide. If you have a very large areola it would be impossible.

If your baby is just sucking on the end of your nipple she won't be getting much milk and your nipples will get sore. In the end, the whole demand and supply circle will stop working. If you are not certain, look at the way she suckles. She should use her whole jaw and you should be able to see the muscle running right up to her ear as it works. The rhythm should be more jerky than a bottle fed baby.

If you don't think she is on right, then put a little finger into the corner of her mouth to break the suction (never just pull off), then touch the corner of her mouth with your nipple so that she turns towards it and opens her mouth. Hold the end of your breast between finger and thumb and make sure the nipple gets right inside.

Latching on often hurts to start with. Once the baby is

actually suckling properly, the 'ouch' fades and you will stop feeling it at all within two weeks or so.

How long should the baby suckle? As long as you both want. It is useless to do it according to a timetable as every baby feeds differently and you may be taking her off before she has had enough to eat (which can lead to sore nipples as well as a hungry baby and dwindling milk supply) or forcing her to suck when she has finished.

Once your baby has been drinking and swallowing (not just sucking and playing) for at least ten minutes on each side, she has probably had enough to drink, so you could try slipping your breast out, if you are getting fed up. If she wants more, she can always have a second course.

How often should you feed your baby? Let your baby set the pace. If you offer her milk whenever she cries for it you will probably have plenty of milk and a pretty contented baby. Some women will happily continue this pattern for as long as their baby wants to suckle. If you find that this constant demand irritates you then you can try to modify your baby's requirements once you have a good supply of milk.

If she is really only interested in sucking, or just feels thirsty, an alternative such as a dummy or a little diluted juice in a bottle could bridge the gap. Use pure fruit juice. Baby drinks such as Delrosa and Ribena may rot your baby's teeth before they arrive. If you can persuade your baby, gradually, to fill up every four hours rather than snack every two hours, you might be able to grab a little space for yourself.

Beware, though, if your baby is suckling frequently because she has just grown a bit and needs more milk, you will find that you are cutting into that vital circle of demand and supply. A baby who has happily managed on four-hour feeds and suddenly demands constant feeding is probably hungry. Give her a couple of days to feed as often as she wants, and you will probably find that your supply builds up and she gradually drops back to more spaced feeds.

Feeding problems

If you have difficulty establishing breastfeeding you may benefit most from some simple, practical help from another mother. Some midwives are very good at showing women how to feed. If yours is not, contact the National Childbirth Trust, to find the name of your nearest breastfeeding counsellor. See page 204.

Flat or inverted nipples won't necessarily cause problems. A baby can latch on to almost any nipple with a bit of patience (see 1 below) and pull it into the right shape by suckling.

If this seems impossibly difficult, try wearing a Woolwich shell (from a clinic, chemist or the hospital) for half an hour before feeds so that your nipple is standing up enough for the baby to latch on to. Once she has got the idea, you should be able to dispense with the shells.

Sore nipples can put you right off but it is important to persevere because the tenderness will soon go and you will start to enjoy it. Here are some tips to help you avoid the problem:

1 Make sure your baby is well latched on (see above).
2 Let her suckle as long and as frequently as she wants. If she is ravenous, she will suck harder and that hurts more.
3 Keep your nipples dry. It is not necessary to wash before and after every feed because you will remove the natural lubricant which protects your nipples. Just rinse in plain water twice a day. Don't use waterproof breast pads which trap the moisture in. Try to spend some time each day with your breasts exposed to the air and wear a cotton bra if you need one.

Many women find that, in spite of all this, they still get tender nipples in the first couple of weeks. If this happens, try:

* A little Massé cream or even Lipsalve around the place where the darker areola meets the breast. Don't cover the nipple itself or you may block the ducts.
* Rotersept spray is preferred by many women. It is an antiseptic in a propellant which is cold and slightly anaesthetises your nipples. The antiseptic may possibly protect you against the bacteria which, in a hospital, may cause mastitis. Most women use it because, sprayed on a couple of minutes before feeding, it seems to take the 'ouch' out of that first mouthful.
* Dry your nipples with a hairdryer after feeding and washing and go topless as much as possible.
* Change the baby's position at the breast, tucking her under your arm to change the position of her mouth.
* A soft flexible nipple shield may help if the nipple gets cracked. The hospital should provide them or you can get them from the National Childbirth Trust or a good chemist.

* Try putting the baby on the less sore breast first and, if the second one still hurts, you could express the milk and give it in a bottle.
* An electric breast pump can be hired from the National Childbirth Trust if a cracked nipple gets worse or leads to infection. (See mastitis, below)

Engorged breasts are hot, hard, and swollen. Engorgement may happen whenever you go without feeding your baby for longer than usual, or for example, if you feed twice on the same side and leave one breast full. Many women get engorged on the third or fourth day when their milk comes in. If you have allowed your baby to suckle frequently on previous days, it may not happen.

If your breasts are full of milk, the best thing you can do is let a little out to ease them. A hot bath, or hot flannels, will help and while you are applying the heat, express a little milk, as we describe on page 167. If there are any painful areas, be sure to stroke the milk out of them. You have a slightly blocked gland (possibly from a tight bra) and if the milk isn't emptied out, it could lead to mastitis.

Mastitis is a breast infection which can occur when an engorged breast becomes infected. You will notice an inflamed red patch on a breast and may feel feverish.

The first treatment is to empty your breast. This will avoid a more serious infection. Follow the same treatment as for engorgement and contact your doctor. You may need antibiotic treatment for the infection. Don't stop feeding your baby, but watch out for thrush (see nappy rash, page 172).

If you are in hospital you may be asked to stop feeding your baby while the infection is treated (it can spread very fast in a hospital). In this case, ask for a breast pump so that you can keep emptying your breast, both as a treatment and to keep up your supply.

Insufficient milk may worry you but, if your baby is alert when awake, wets at least six or eight nappies a day, and produces bright yellow or greenish nappies when she needs to (see page 170), then she is unlikely to be starving so you can forget the scales.

If she wants to suck all the time, it could be that she is hungry but maybe she just likes to suck. See if a dummy will give you a little time off.

If your previously full breasts seem soft and smaller (at about six weeks) this does not mean they are empty. You are just beginning to adjust to each other and produce the right amount. If one breast produces more than the other, it won't affect the total amount.

If you are really concerned about your milk production, you can increase your production by allowing the baby to suckle as often as she is able to. Generally speaking, a breastfeeding woman who is eating a good diet (see page 179), drinking as much as her body tells her she needs, and getting a reasonable amount of rest should be able to produce enough milk to feed her baby. There is no reason why breastfeeding should not be part of normal life and normal pursuits.

However, if you feel that your production is not as high as you would like, take twenty-four hours out of your normal life. Get your partner, mother, sister or a friend to take over everything else for a day (including cooking you tempting and nutritious meals) and spend the time alone with your baby allowing her to suckle as often as she can. You can even wake her occasionally and see if she will latch on. The more your breasts are stimulated, the more they will produce. If you are relaxed and not fighting against your baby's needs, the milk message will get through.

It's time to think again about breast-feeding when it starts to take over your life and make you miserable. Norma said;

'My first baby was no trouble at all but Ben was a real handful. He was never really content. He didn't drop off to sleep after a feed but squirmed all the way through and then cried for more as soon as I put him down. I was exhausted and finding it hard to cope. Finally my husband suggested putting him on the bottle so that we could at least share the burden. With David taking a bigger share I was at last able to relax and start to enjoy my baby.'

Sharing the load

Occasional bottle feeds will not affect your milk supply if they are managed carefully, and not introduced until breastfeeding is well-established. Sucking from a teat is so different from suckling that, if your baby starts feeding from a bottle in the first few days, she may refuse to feed from the breast. Once she has realised that there is more to a breast than food, it is very unlikely that she will prefer a bottle to you.

On the other hand, a baby who has never had to suck from a teat may refuse point blank to do so when, at a later date, you want to leave her with someone else for a few hours. Unless you are prepared to take her with you everywhere until she is at least six months old, it is a good idea to give her occasional drinks of cool water in a bottle (boil both for five minutes) or expressed breast milk so that she knows how to suck.

It is wise to avoid even the occasional cow's milk feed at least in the first four months if you want to avoid allergies. You can either express and bottle your own milk (see section on expressing) or buy a formula made from soy protein isolate. Many of the formula manufacturers now produce soy-based ones (see page 167).

Never use formula to supplement your own feeds if you want to keep up your milk supply. If your baby is fed from a bottle while you are out, you should express that feed by hand, to avoid getting painfully engorged and to keep up the demand on your own milk supply.

Regular bottle feeds can be built into an established breastfeeding schedule if you have to go back to work, or want to share the care of your child with someone else. Then if you make sure that the bottle feed is given regularly, at the same time every day, your milk supply will soon adjust to this pattern and you won't fill up so much. If you want to maintain your own supply for any length of time, you must make sure that your baby feeds from you frequently, in the time that you are together.

Shared feeding   Some women who have chosen to live together with their babies or who have made friends through a postnatal group feed each other's babies to give each other a break. Of course, many women find the idea rather odd, if not positively disgusting, but it has a great deal to recommend it:

'I had never planned to do it but, faced with this howling, thirsty infant who didn't know one end of a bottle from the other, it seemed crazy not to. Here was I with breasts full of milk and there she was desperate for it. It was rather odd at first, a bit like cuddling up to your best friend's lover, but she didn't seem to notice the difference so I relaxed and let her get on with it. At least she wasn't crying any more. When her mum came back she didn't mind a bit, in fact I think she felt

a bit cheated that she didn't get the opportunity to do the same for mine.'

Expressing milk   Make sure you are comfortable and relaxed so that your let down reflex will work. It may help to do it after a hot bath or to bathe your breast with warm flannels. Then hold your breast in one hand and stroke down with the other, squeezing the milk ducts behind the nipple as you stroke. If you stroke, squeeze and then let go, in a gentle rhythm, you should find that the milk squirts out in a stream.

If hand expressing yields only a few drops, and a sore breast, try an expressor. A Kaneson which looks rather like a bicycle pump in reverse works pretty well. You can buy them in large chemists or from the National Childbirth Trust (see page 204).

If you want to keep the milk and feed your baby with it, you must ensure that the pump and bottle are sterilised. Once your milk is outside you, hygiene must be as strict as that for any bottle-feeding mother (see page 173). You can collect an ounce or two after each feed over a twenty-four hour period if you store the container in the fridge. If you want to keep the milk longer than that it must be frozen. It will last for a week in the ice compartment of your fridge and for three months in a freezer.

If you are expressing milk for a baby in special care, or because of mastitis, the hospital should provide an electric pump. If you are at home, you can hire one from the National Childbirth Trust (see page 204).

Extra milk can be donated to a milk bank for other babies. Mention it to your midwife or health visitor.

Bottle-feeding

Your baby is not getting the protection of antibodies from you with which to fight infection so you must be particularly careful to avoid introducing germs. This means maintaining scrupulous hygiene (see page 173).

Equipment should include at least eight bottles if you intend to bottle-feed completely. If you are only giving an occasional feed, one or two will do.

A bucket with a lid will do as a steriliser, or a large covered saucepan if you intend to boil rather than using steriliser tablets or liquid. If you use a bucket, you don't need to fill it full each time – put in the right quantity to cover everything and then hold it all down with a plate.

A bottle brush should be used for washing milk out.

Formula can be bought at your local baby clinic slightly cheaper than at the shops. Ask your midwife or health visitor for advice on which feed to use. If you are concerned about allergies, you may prefer to use a soy formula. It is slightly more expensive than ordinary formula, but if you have a family history of allergy your doctor may be prepared to give you a prescription.

You must always follow the instructions on the packet extremely carefully and never add extra powder to thicken the feed. Your baby cannot cope with the extra minerals she will be swallowing so she will get very thirsty and demand more food. Eventually she could get seriously ill.

Teat hole size If it is too big, your baby may choke or bring her feed straight back. If it is too small, she may struggle for ages, obviously hungry, but making no impression on the milk. Try the tipping test. Milk should drip out steadily but shouldn't stream out.

How often should you feed? Let your baby set the pattern. If you have made up a day's feeds and left them in the fridge, you should be able to feed her whenever she seems hungry. If the weather is very hot and she is feeding often, you could try giving her cooled, boiled water, occasionally. Your baby will drink the milk at room temperature if she is used to it. Take the chill off it by all means but it doesn't have to be the same temperature as breast milk. In fact, it is much less likely to harbour germs if it is not warmed.

Feed your baby as though you were breastfeeding. Hold her close so that she feels safe and warm and can hear your heartbeat. Never prop the bottle in a cot or pram as she may choke on it.

Tilt the bottle so that the teat is always full of milk to avoid the baby gulping air. If she doesn't cotton on that she should let go every few sucks to let some air in, gently detach her. If she keeps sucking she will create a vacuum and nothing will come out. Some bottles come with detachable milk bags which collapse as the milk goes out, avoiding these problems.

Wind

We worry a great deal about wind in this country though it doesn't seem to bother other babies half so much. You do not

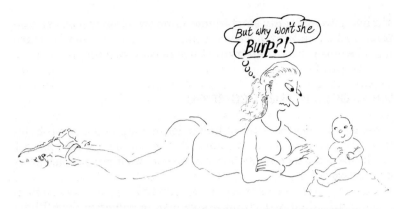

If wind isn't worrying your baby, don't let it worry you.

have to go through a ritual to get wind up. At the end of a feed, it is a good idea to hold your baby upright, against your shoulder for a few minutes to allow any air in her stomach to bubble up. If after a few minutes nothing has happened and she wants to sleep, just lie her down on her tummy. The pressure on her tummy will help the wind to find its way out the other end.

If your baby seems to be in pain shortly after a feed, try giving her a few sips of cooled peppermint tea or peppermint essence diluted in cooled boiled water.

Babies' tummies can give trouble in the first three months. Just do what you would do for yourself: hold her against a warm firm surface (your shoulder) and stroke her back. If problems continue, read the section on colic (page 190). If wind isn't worrying your baby, don't let it worry you.

Introducing other foods

There is no rush to start solid foods. In the first four months, your baby will have trouble digesting anything other than milk. Most of the other food will simply go straight through. If your baby is sensitive you may also find that you are actually triggering off an allergy (such as eczema) which could have been avoided if you had waited to introduce solids at a later date.

If your baby is content and gaining weight on milk alone, don't bother to start introducing solids until around six months.

If a big baby suddenly starts demanding two-hourly feeds at, say, three month and three weeks, you may prefer, cautiously, starting on solids rather than trying to increase your own milk supply.

WHAT GOES IN MUST COME OUT

A healthy baby wets at least half a dozen nappies a day, probably more. She may dirty that many also in the first weeks though gradually a pattern will emerge of one or two dirty nappies every day or two.

In the first two or three days your baby will produce sticky black stuff called meconium. As your milk comes in it will have a soupy consistency and turn green and then bright yellow. If you are bottle-feeding, it will be slightly lighter in colour and bulkier.

What is not normal?

Breastfed babies may dirty one nappy once a week, or every nappy. Both are normal. Bottle-fed babies should have at least one dirty nappy a day.

Constipation in breastfed babies is most unlikely. If your bottle-fed baby misses a couple of days, ask your health visitor for advice.

Diarrhoea is more common but quite difficult to identify. Babies produce pretty liquid stuff normally. If she has mucus in it, if it smells unpleasant, or seems very watery, she may have an upset tummy. If you are breastfeeding, just keep feeding as much as your baby wants. If your baby is on bottles, dilute them by half as much boiled water again for a day to try and wash any bacteria out. She may want to suck more often this way but it will be good for her to get more liquid. See page 183 for when to call a doctor.

Nappies

Nappies can be folded a number of ways. Here is one method for newborn babies (see illustration on page 171).

Tie plastic pants are best for small babies. The method shown

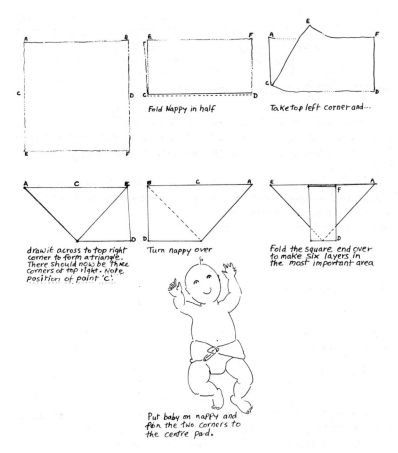

Fold Nappy in half

Take top left corner and...

draw it across to top right corner to form a triangle. There should now be three corners at top right. Note position of point 'c'.

Turn nappy over

Fold the square end over to make six layers in the most important area

Put baby on nappy and pin the two corners to the centre pad.

for tying them can also be used for pads on newborn babies (see illustration on page 172).

Change your baby before or after feeds and when she is dirty or very wet. If your baby has a delicate skin which is prone to nappy rash, you may need to change her more often than this.

Avoid changing during *your* sleeping time unless she is wet through or dirty. Plenty of padding and fabric Ever Dri liners (available from Mothercare or Boots) should see your baby through the night.

There is never any need to wake a sleeping baby just to change her nappy.

Clean the area between the legs very carefully at each change. Use plain warm water and then pat dry.

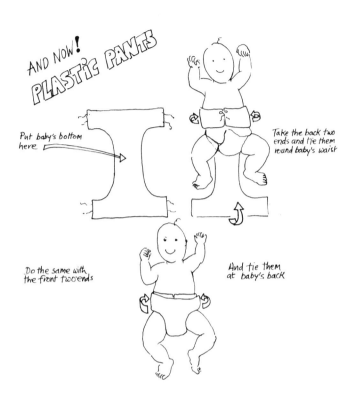

AND NOW! PLASTIC PANTS

Put baby's bottom here

Take the back two ends and tie them round baby's waist

Do the same with the front two ends

And tie them at baby's back

Nappy rash can attack even the most carefully kept baby. Your baby's skin type and vulnerability to allergy is as significant as the number of times you bath and change her.

One of the first signs of impending nappy rash may be a strong smell of ammonia in her nappies. This means that the bacteria, which cause rashes, are at work. Check your sterilising techniques (see pages 173–4) and make sure the bacteria have been cleared.

If your baby shows signs of redness, keep her as dry as possible. Leave her without a nappy for as long as possible, use one-way liners or all-in-one disposables and leave her without any plastic pants for as long as you can.

Zinc and castor oil smoothed on a dry bottom and in all the crevices will help to make her skin water-resistant. Some babies are allergic to zinc so watch out for that. A cream called *Metanium* usually works like magic to clear up any redness.

If the rash persists, check for allergies. Leave out the water softener when you wash nappies and make sure they are very well rinsed. Avoid bathing the baby in detergent and soap, use plain warm water. Check with your doctor that she hasn't got thrush (a fungal infection which usually shows up as little white bits in her mouth). Thrush should certainly be suspected if the rash causes discomfort and crying.

HYGIENE

In a world where water comes clean out of the taps and human waste goes straight into an efficient sewerage system, it is not immediately obvious why babies need so much protection from bacteria.

In fact, your hygienic world is full of bacteria; it is just that your body has grown used to the particular bugs which you meet each day. Your baby, fresh out of a sterile womb, has had no opportunity to adjust to your normal level of bacteria. Just as you may fall ill with a tummy bug on a foreign trip when the people who actually live there are perfectly healthy, your baby may fall ill when exposed to germs which your body can fight quite easily.

This doesn't mean that you should keep her from having any contact with germs. If she is to build up resistance to bacteria, she must be exposed to them – gradually. So you needn't worry if a rattle falls off the cot on to the carpet and then goes back into her mouth, but you should avoid putting a rattle that has fallen in the road back into her mouth.

Bottles, teats and all the equipment used for making up feeds should be sterilised. Otherwise milk will collect in the crevices and bacteria will multiply.

To sterilise your bottles, first wash them well using a bottle brush and clean the inside of the teats carefully. Then, if you are using sterilising tablets or liquid in a tank, read the instructions very carefully. Make up the steriliser, ensure that the bottles are full of the liquid and that everything is kept under the water with a floating lid or plate.

Five minutes' hard boiling will do just as well. Use a pan with a lid to ensure that any exposed bits are sterilised in the steam.

Before taking the bottles out wash your hands, and avoid

touching the top of the teat. The sterilant must not be washed off before you give the bottle to the baby.

Spoons used for giving water or medicine to a baby of less than four months should be sterilised as bottles are.

Dummies are always dropping but don't use ribbon to tie them on as that could be dangerous. If a dummy falls in the cot or pram, don't worry. If it falls on the street or a dirty floor, don't give it back. Keep some spare sterilised ones with you.

Nappies should be sterilised before washing. Even if you don't wash them every day, you should change the steriliser in the bucket daily to make sure that it is capable of killing any bacteria in the nappies. It is this bacteria which causes nappy rash. If your baby's nappies have an ammonia smell about them, you may not be sterilising them properly.

Make sure that you rinse out every trace of the sterilant and be cautious about using a softener. Both can irritate the skin.

You don't really need to wash wet nappies that have been sterilised. If you can be bothered to keep them separate, you can simply rinse the wet ones and wash the soiled ones.

Clothes, even if they have been wet and soiled, do not need to be sterilised. Just wash them. The bacteria causing nappy rash is only a problem when it is trapped next to the baby's skin in a nice warm damp environment.

Floors and furniture don't need to be sterile! Make sure that odd bits of food are not left near enough for your baby to get hold of and eat. If you get pee on the floor it isn't a health hazard, just mop it up. If it's the other stuff use a little antiseptic to get rid of the bacteria.

Pets carry germs so don't let your cat walk on any surface where you may prepare food. Keep pets out of the cot, and don't let them lick your baby's face.

Bathing need not be done every day. You should wipe the baby's face with warm, dampened cotton wool and sponge her bottom and between her legs with mild soap and rinse well with warm water at least daily. Make sure that you do this in a warm room and then pat her dry quickly afterwards so that she does not get chilled.

Chapter 7

PARENTHOOD

HOW DO YOU FEEL?

Up

'I have never, in my whole life, felt as happy as I did in those first days home. The three of us floated through the day on a cloud of exhausted bliss. Friends visited bringing food with them, cards poured in, and the flat was filled with flowers. I have never felt so loved.'

A birth is a special event. However much alone you may have felt during pregnancy, you will almost certainly find that, once the baby is there, people will rally round. Crusty fathers who disapprove of the baby, its father, or you, suddenly remember how to smile; friends nip in just to peer into the recesses of the cot and coo; it isn't just the baby which makes it so exciting, it's the event itself.

If you are exhausted by attention, make yourself a 'no visitors' time of day, or hang a notice on the door and take the phone off the hook when you get a chance to sleep.

Down

The euphoria of the first days is a fragile feeling. It is fed on love and attention from the people around you but it can quite easily spin itself around. Your new responsibility may seem frightening. Advice from well-meaning friends and relatives may confuse you. The mixture of anxiety and mood changes takes some women down rather than up.

Postnatal depression is a word which can be very badly used. A real depression is more than just a feeling of sadness. If you feel exhausted rather than exhilarated and quite unable to cope with the unaccustomed isolation or the strain of a second baby in addition to an energetic toddler, you are not ill. Nor are you 'making a fuss', 'inadequate' or a 'bad mother'. You probably just need a bit of mothering yourself.

If she lives close enough talk to your own mother about it. You won't want her to take over, but if you ask her to help, and make it clear where the division lies, you will probably find her a loving tower of strength. If this is impossible, find yourself a temporary mother. A friend with older children, or a postnatal support group may do just as well (see page 191). Remember that most people feel flattered to be asked for help and it may not take much to get you going again.

If the thought of finding someone to talk to just fills you with even more despair, if you are persistently sad, remote, careless, sleeping badly (even when you get the chance) and eating little, you may be more seriously depressed. Even a severe depression is a hurdle which can be overcome with the right help. Your health visitor or a sympathetic GP may be the best bet. Or you could contact Meet a Mum, or the Association for Post Natal Illness which has a telephone counselling service. Either organisation will respond immediately by phone or return post. (See pages 203–4.)

YOUR BODY

The postnatal exam

Six weeks after the birth you should visit your GP or the hospital for a postnatal examination. It should include:
An internal vaginal examination to check the condition of your womb, vagina and muscles;
A smear (cancer) test;
Your tummy will be felt (palpated) to ensure that it is returning to normal;
Your stitch scar should be inspected;
Your breasts may be examined;
Contraception will be discussed, so it is important to consider what you will want.

Contraception

Contraception should be used as soon as you start having intercourse again, even though you may not have any periods for a while. If you wait for your first period you may get pregnant before it arrives.

If you are fully breastfeeding you are less likely to get pregnant because the hormones circulating in your body will not normally allow ovulation. However, some breastfeeding women ovulate again very soon after giving birth so don't take any risks.

Hormonal contraceptives   The combined Pill is not recommended for breastfeeding women because it may suppress your milk and the hormones in it will go straight through the milk to your baby. The mini Pill (progestagen only) is often given in hospitals because it doesn't stop your milk and contains a lower dose of hormones. Nobody really knows whether even this amount of hormone may have an effect on a tiny baby so, if you are intending to use the Pill as your normal contraceptive method, you may prefer to use a sheath for the first six weeks.

An injection of progestagen (Depo-Provera) may also be suggested. The manufacturers now admit that it's best not to use it for the first four to six weeks after delivery. Given at this time it may be responsible for prolonged bleeding and, nobody yet knows what effect it could have on a breastfeeding baby. You should not be given any injections after pregnancy without a clear explanation about what they are for and what they contain.

Intra-uterine contraceptive devices (IUDs) are best left until six weeks after the birth or for three months after a Caesarean.

A cap (diaphragm) should be refitted no sooner than six weeks after the birth. Get the size checked again after three to six months or if you lose or gain weight.

Sheaths are probably the best form of contraception for the first six weeks provided you use plenty of extra lubrication (preferably spermicide) to prevent rubbing against a tender perineum.

Spermicidal foam is not usually recommended for use without a cap or sheath but, if you are fully breastfeeding, your fertility is low anyway, so it could tide you over for the first six weeks. Non-foaming spermicides are unreliable alone.

Sex

Sex may be the last thing on your mind. Some women do feel turned on by the intensity of the experience and the closeness you feel at home together. Others feel that there simply isn't enough emotional room for pleasurable sex or they are just too tired.

If you try having sexual intercourse and find penetration painful it may be that you are still bruised. If the pain persists beyond two months ask your doctor to take a look at your stitch line. It may be that you have picked up a mild infection because the natural balance of your vagina has been upset. This is very easily treated.

It could also be that your stitch line is hypersensitive. If it has been tightly stitched the flesh may have puckered and thickened. Scar tissue is less elastic than undamaged flesh so the entrance may feel tighter than usual. Most of these problems will sort themselves out, given time and patience.

You can help yourself by taking a long, lingering time over sex to make sure that you are relaxed and lubricating properly. You may find that extra lubrication will help now. Hormone changes mean that you are producing less than you normally would. If you are breastfeeding, you may feel grateful for extra help for some time. Use a water soluble lubricant such as KY or spermicidal jelly.

Don't force yourself into sex which hurts. If initial penetration is painful you may freeze up completely and that could set up a psychological pattern which is hard to break. Sex does not have to include penetration to be a pleasure for both of you.

Very occasionally, tight stitching may cause a bigger problem. In this case an operation to cut and restitch may be suggested. You may first prefer to massage your perineum with cream (some women suggest vitamin E cream), do pelvic floor exercises to teach yourself how to relax the area, and plenty of personal exploration with your own fingers. When you do try again, use plenty of extra lubrication.

Some women are concerned because their vaginas feel too loose and they cannot feel the way they used to. The answer to this lies in pelvic floor exercises (see page 8).

Partners can help by being extremely patient. It takes some women many months to recover interest in sex completely. Physical reasons are not the only ones. As one woman put it,

'I felt battered and abused. I couldn't even think about that part of my body without shuddering, for months.'

Looking after yourself

It is very easy to busy yourself with others and totally forget about your own needs. If you are breastfeeding you need to eat well. Your body is providing food for your growing baby as well as you and you need 500 calories per day more than usual to supply both your needs. If you are concerned about your weight, just eat normally, your baby will drink the extra weight away. Look back to chapter 1 (page 2) to remind yourself what a good diet should be. If you are feeling tired and low you may simply be eating badly. Make a special effort to eat foods rich in vitamin B (wholemeal bread, green vegetables, whole cereals), plenty of protein foods (cheese, beans, meat) and cut down on sugar. Drink pure fruit juices to provide vitamin C, and plenty of water. Breastfeeding is thirsty work. Your thirst will tell you how much liquid you need.

RED TAPE

Registration

The hospital will notify the local registry office within thirty-six hours of the birth. You then have six weeks (three in Scotland) to think of a name and register the birth.

If you are married, either you or your husband may register the birth.

If you are not married, you may give your baby any name you like (without permission), but you may not put the father's name on the registration form, as the father, without his permission (unless you have an affiliation order from a court).

This means that, if you want both names to go on the register, you must both go to the office. Failing that the father must either sign a *statutory declaration* for you to take, giving permission for you to register his name (check with a law centre or citizen's advice bureau); or you can go together, at a later date, and add his name.

The father cannot insist on having his name on the registration form without your consent.

The birth certificate may be short (including only the baby's name) or long (including both the parent's names). The longer version costs more.

Employment rights

Your employment rights could be endangered if you do not carry out your legal obligations. Your employer may write to you, not earlier than seven weeks after the expected date of the birth, to ask whether you intend to return to work. YOU MUST REPLY WITHIN FOURTEEN DAYS or you could lose your right to the job. Re-read the section on maternity rights (page 72).

Money

Child benefit is paid for every child under the age of 16. Claim by filling in form CH2 and index slip CH3 from any social security office. If you are a single parent you may claim a special allowance on claim form CH11a. Send the birth certificate with the form.

Tax allowances will not change if you are married but, if you are not, you may claim an extra allowance which is equivalent in size to the married man's tax allowance. This allowance may be claimed by whoever has day-to-day care of the child or it can be split between carers.

Unemployment benefit or supplementary benefit claimants are eligible for an extra allowance for the baby. If you are a single parent claiming supplementary benefit, the Department of Health and Social Services (DHSS) may ask for the father's name in order to serve an 'affiliation order' and get him to pay you an allowance. You do not have to give his name if you don't want to, though if it is on the birth registration, you won't be able to keep it from them.

Regular maintenance payments from the father will be deducted automatically from your supplementary benefit. If the father does not pay regularly it may be better to sign over your affiliation order to the DHSS so that they make sure you get the right money every week.

Prescription and dental charges are not made for another year.

YOUR BABY

'The baby does totally change your life. I went into shock after about two weeks when I suddenly realised that I had no control of my life any more. The baby wakes when he wants to, even when I am tired. I am terrified that something may happen to him and yet, after five nights without sleep, I am even more terrified of my own temper. There are days when I just don't want to be a mother any more.'

Every new mother has periods of anxiety about her baby and her life which, six months later, may seem strangely obsessive. Every change is cause for alarm: the first rash appears and you are sure it's the plague; you creep in while she sleeps to make sure she is still breathing.

Who can help?

A midwife will have responsibility for you and your baby for the first ten days (or a month if either of you have had problems). She will come daily to see that you are well and give advice about practical problems and baby care. You may feel that some of your worries are too silly to waste time with but, if they are worrying you, they are part of your midwife's job.

A health visitor should take over from the midwife on the tenth day. The health visitor will not visit regularly unless you have particular problems but she should give you her name and tell you where she can be contacted. She is a trained nurse who has done a special course and now works entirely in the community looking after the health of mothers and children. Her job is to advise you and give you the practical help you need. Get to know your health visitor, she can be a good friend to you, as Suzanne discovered:

'My children were 3½ years and four months. The house was terrible: unplastered walls, no hot water in the kitchen, and we were heavily in debt. Then my husband left.
One day I found myself throwing a cup of tea at the kids.

Then I just managed to stop myself throwing my baby on the floor. I was frightened enough to ring my health visitor, but I was scared she would take them into care. She said that all I needed was a break and got two afternoons in a nursery for the children. I felt so forgiven.'

Handicapped babies may require extra attention. Your health visitor and doctor should advise you of the facilities available. You can ask your GP to refer you to a paediatrician (child specialist) who can explain your child's particular problems and how you can best help yourself and her. If you are not happy with the advice you are given you can ask your GP for a referral to the district assessment centre or the hospital paediatric department.

The local social services department can give you the name of local branches of those organisations concerned with the particular handicap your baby is suffering from and of any local parents group where you can share ideas and give each other support. Of course all the usual facilities are open to you as well. Your child and the other children will benefit from each other's company as they get older.

Well baby clinics weigh babies regularly, give routine immunisation and developmental checks and advise you on any practical problems. Your health visitor should give you the address and the times of clinics when she visits you.

Immunisation

When your baby is three months old you will be asked to have her immunised against diphtheria, tetanus, polio and whooping cough.

Immunisation has virtually wiped out the infectious diseases which used to be childhood killers, but lately controversy has arisen over whooping cough vaccination. If your baby is susceptible to fits you would be better to avoid this vaccination (discuss it with your doctor). You can still get the others done.

From the point of view of society as a whole, it is better that most children should be vaccinated because the problem of death and disablement from the disease by far outweighs the small number of children who have suffered brain damage from whooping cough vaccine.

For the individual parent the argument is not simple. As Sheila said,

'I had waited so long for a baby, now here she is healthy and happy. How could I take even the tiniest risk by getting her vaccinated. I will just make sure she doesn't come into contact with other children who could have whooping cough.'

Her fears are understandable but every parent who chooses to protect their own child against vaccination side effects without a specific health reason is putting the whole vaccination programme at risk. Vaccination will only cut down disease if virtually everyone is vaccinated so that there is no possibility of passing it on to newborn babies who are the most vulnerable.

Side effects Your baby may become feverish. A small dose of Calpol or Panadol Elixir will soon make her comfortable enough to sleep it off.

However, if she becomes floppy, irritable, or has slight 'fits' you should contact your doctor. This may be evidence of a reaction to whooping cough vaccine and it could be a reason to avoid the second dose.

Homeopathy is a branch of medicine which is based on different principles from orthodox medicine. Homeopaths provide a kind of immunisation against whooping cough which is much milder in its effect (see page 203).

WHEN TO CALL A DOCTOR

Remember, you are your baby's best monitor. If you feel that she is suddenly different from usual: lethargic, pale, quiet and off her food, or her crying seems more insistent than usual and is accompanied by other symptoms such as ear rubbing, vomiting, or a rash, get a doctor's advice. Baby illnesses can blow up quickly and it is better to be on the safe side.

Vomiting is pretty common in young babies. Most babies bring back a little milk after a meal. Even if she appears to bring back most of it you needn't worry provided that it doesn't occur several times in a row and it isn't accompanied by diarrhoea, feverishness, or a rash. If she appears grey and limp, consult your doctor even if there are no other symptoms.

Diarrhoea is not easy to identify in a young baby. If it seems particularly watery or contains mucus she may have a slight infection and you should see a doctor if it persists. If it is accompanied by vomiting, feverishness, loss of appetite, or crying or if she seems generally unwell, then consult your doctor straight away. If you are breastfeeding it is very unlikely to be serious. If your baby is on a bottle it is wise to be cautious about upset tummies.

Temperatures, with no other symptoms, are not likely to be serious. Just take off a layer of clothing, and if necessary sponge her down with warm water. (Make sure the room is warm enough so that she doesn't get chilled.) A baby with a temperature can get convulsions if she is allowed to get too hot.

Give her Calpol or Panadol Elixir if she doesn't respond or, if the fever lasts more than twenty-four hours, you should then call your doctor.

If there are other symptoms, such as a strange cry, limpness, vomiting, sickness, or anything else, you should contact your doctor without delay. If you are in doubt ring anyway, you will only worry more if you don't.

Colds are hard to avoid but rarely more than a nuisance. A slight fever is not unusual, but if she also seems lethargic, her breathing sounds tight and rasping, or she has a hard dry cough, contact your doctor just to make sure she has not got a chest infection.

Falls If she cries lustily, she is probably all right. If it is a bad fall get your doctor just to check her over. If she seems quiet, or falls into a deep sleep shortly after, consult your doctor. If she is unconscious, call an ambulance.

In general, contact your doctor when you are worried, and again if the condition changes unexpectedly. You can take the baby to the doctor, it saves delay and the doctor's time.

SAFETY

Babies need to be free to explore as soon as they are able to but that means a great deal of care and vigilance from parents and other caretakers. In a simpler society it may be possible for a child to learn about danger through experience but experiencing an electric socket or gas cooker might rule out future experiences altogether. The best way to protect your baby is to ensure that her world is as safe as you can make it. These are some of the hazards to watch for.

Suffocation is a danger if you give your baby a pillow or draw up the string round the end of a sleeping bag.

Cats should be kept out of the cot by use of a cat net, or simply shutting the door.

Scalding is best avoided by always putting the cold water into the bath first so that you can never put her accidentally into a hot bath. Practise putting tea and coffee cups out of reach and in the middle of the table, and avoid tablecloths which can be tugged.

Bumpers round the inside of a cot stop a small baby from getting its head stuck in the bars. Never fit a harness on a cot.

Toddlers can be a hazard to new babies but, though a watchful eye is sensible, don't let the toddler know that you are nervous. An over enthusiastic hug may knock your baby over but it probably won't hurt her. If you descend vengefully on the older child you can be pretty certain that next time she will get her own back by actually trying to inflict damage.

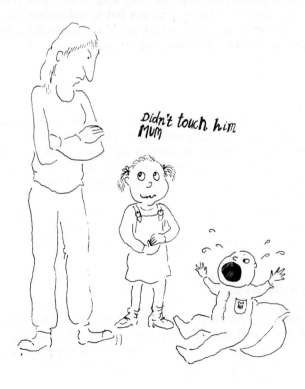

Beads, peanuts, screws and similar small objects are a danger to babies who automatically put everything in their mouths. Peanuts are particularly dangerous because they can be inhaled and get stuck in the windpipe and the peanut oil can destroy lung tissue. If you have an older child who plays with Lego or other small objects try and create a special place for these toys. You can explain that the baby will otherwise spoil her games.

Car travel for a small baby should be in a carrycot held down with a safety strap. If you have the baby on your knee it is against the law to sit in front.

Hot or cold A small baby cannot regulate her own temperature very easily so you have to be very careful to ensure that she is neither overwrapped nor underwrapped. Both can be dangerous. Except for short trips, you should try to keep your baby in a warm atmosphere (not less than 65°F), then, make sure she is wearing just one more layer than you are. If the back of her neck or chest seems cool, add more clothing, if she seems clammy, flushed and fretting, she may be too hot so take some off. Don't leave her in direct sunshine which could burn her delicate skin. Do make sure she is reasonably cool on a very hot day.

SLEEP

Most child care books suggest that, at about six weeks, your baby will start to sleep through the night. They probably want to be optimistic. A great many babies do not sleep through the night for many months and, surveys have shown that something like 14 per cent are still disturbing their parents at the age of 3. We know from experience!

If you know that this is possible, it will help you to see the question of lost sleep as a long-term problem which you will have to come to terms with, rather than a brief inconvenience.

Setting a pattern

Babies differ in the amount of sleep they need. What they miss at night, they will make up during the day. If your baby wants very little sleep there is not much you can do about it. She is not suffering, though you might be. As she gets a little older, you can help to shape her sleeping periods so that the bulk of her sleeping time coincides with your needs. If you work during the day you may want to encourage a late bedtime so that you spend the evenings together. If you cherish your evenings and don't mind an early start to the day you can pull bedtime back earlier. One habit you will want to instil from the start is sleeping through the night.

Mark the difference between night and day. Keep her with you during the daytime and keep night-time contact to the minimum: don't change her unless she is dirty or sodden, keep the light low, wrap her well if she sleeps better that way, and lie her on her tummy so she doesn't wake herself with flailing limbs. Where she sleeps may make all the difference to how you sleep.

In your bed?
Nicky's first child was born 15 years ago when babies were fed four-hourly and left to cry between feeds. By three months she slept through the night and never a peep has been heard since. But Nicky found the experience very distressing. Her third baby, Reuben, is now 4. He stayed in her bed from birth:

'I didn't really lose any sleep because he was with me. At about three months he seemed to want more space so I put him into a cot. Some people worry that they will squash the baby but why should they? You don't fall out of bed unless you are drugged or drunk, so why should you roll over on your baby?'

If you do take your baby into your bed you must accept the possibility of company for some time to come, or go through what may be a difficult weaning process at a later stage. Reuben still wakes and comes into their bed most nights.

If you are lucky the sheer satisfaction of this early experience will encourage your baby to recognise the difference between night and day and get used to sleeping soundly even when you move her to a separate room.

Of course you may have a wriggly baby who won't let you sleep even if she is snoring. In this case you will probably have to try something else.

Out of the room

If you are determined not to let your baby into your bed it may
be better to move her right out of your room. Particularly if she
is a first baby and you wake with her every snuffle. Your rest-
lessness may disturb her too. If she is out of the room and you
cannot wake each other you might well find that she sleeps more
soundly.

Of course, if this doesn't work you will then find yourself
with cold trips down the corridor rather than a step across the
room.

Being firm

If, by the time your baby is three or four months old, you are
still not getting a decent night's sleep, you may have to get tough.
By this time you can be fairly sure that she is waking through
habit, not through hunger. You should now be able to persuade
her that nights are not for eating. Breastfed babies are particularly likely to go on waking just because they enjoy those cosy
moments. If you gradually withdraw the pleasure your baby may
not bother to wake any more.

You could try replacing feeds during your sleeping time with
a bottle of milk and water and then gradually reducing contact
at night to a comforting stroke. You may find that your baby is
pretty angry if her mother goes in and then doesn't give her the
breast. She will probably just fight until you give in. If your
partner can take over late night feeds, the process of withdrawal
will probably be quicker.

You will hate it, your partner will be exhausted, every night
will seem like a week, but if you stick at it, you will probably
find that, within a week or two, your baby will give up waking
at night. This technique can be used at any age but with older
babies it may take longer.

If this doesn't work, or you have no one to share the nights
with, you may have to take an even firmer line. Julia was alone
with five-month-old twins so she didn't have the luxury of mud-
dling through. She felt she just had to be able to sleep at night:

*'My mum came to stay for a few days and that gave me moral
support. Then I just put them to bed at 7 p.m. and left them
crying for ten minutes. I used to sit outside the room with a
watch and wait. If after ten minutes they seemed to be getting
quieter then I would leave them a little longer. I did the same*

thing if they woke during the night. It was agony but within a week it had worked. They slept and didn't disturb me and we were all much happier and more energetic during the day.'

These techniques are remarkably effective if you carry them out consistently and compensate with plenty of love and cuddles during the day.

If you work away from home during the day you may feel that, although you don't want a disturbed night, you cannot bear to be tough with a baby who you only see at weekends, and in the evening. Many parents in this situation, who have resolved never to let their babies into bed, have decided that three in a bed is in fact a better solution than sleepless nights. A second mattress in her room may give you an alternative if you find this too crowded. It helps to get the baby to sleep in her own bed initially to give you some privacy and togetherness. Then when she wakes in the early hours, you can take it in turns to sleep with her.

Emergency measures

If nothing seems to work and you are running ragged, you can speak to your doctor about giving your baby something to make her sleep. You may find that if your baby responds to sleeping mixture (they don't all respond) you can grab a couple of nights' sleep. You can't rely on drugs as a long-term solution because, not only are they bad for your baby, they also stop being effective.

Hyperactivity

Some babies appear to get by on less sleep than the average adult. First check with your doctor that she is not suffering from some allergy which makes her wakeful. If not, she may adapt to spending time alone in her cot if you make sure it is safe, with plenty to do and look at, and a night light. (See page 203.)

Going to sleep

Some babies just hate to close their eyes in the evening. They need rocking and soothing and stroking and feeding before they will finally let go.

A baby who yells fretfully all evening may actually be overtired. Try setting up a bedtime routine and then just putting her down in her cot and leaving her. She will probably yell for five minutes and then fall asleep. Overtired babies often cry themselves to sleep and it will do them no harm.

Linda has three children:

'With the first I was up and down all night, rocking him and walking the corridors. By the time I had the third, I knew I could just put her down and leave her. She got used to it from the start and hasn't been any trouble unless she has been ill. She is a contented, happy baby.'

You could try leaving a radio on softly outside her room so that she doesn't feel left out and see whether she is happier with or without a night light.

Colic

This is a mysterious ailment which bothers some babies. It usually disappears by three months but that can feel like three years. A colicky baby cries as if in pain for long periods of time, and cannot be consoled for more than a few minutes either by feeding or by cuddling. These crying bouts often occur in the evening, and the most useful thing you can do is try and share the burden. A baby with colic is sometimes calmed by constant motion. You and your partner can take turns walking her in a baby sling. If you are a single parent, you may find that a friend or relative will be prepared to give you occasional breaks if they understand the problem. Your doctor may also prescribe a drug called Merbentyl which sometimes helps.

Don't assume that your baby has colic just because she cries in the evening. Many babies are dreadful at this time. It may be because you are tired and your milk supply is low at this time, or your baby is overtired (see above).

Constant crying can make even the most saintly parent feel violent. If you do feel like this then put her in her cot, close the door, and get as far away as you can from the noise until you feel calm again. You won't be able to comfort her if you feel tense and angry, so ten minutes spent doing relaxation exercises will be more useful to both of you than ten more minutes going out of your mind.

You could explore the possibility of allergies: switch a

bottle-fed baby to a soy formula and, if you breastfeed, try cutting allergens such as cows' milk from your own diet.

KEEPING YOUR HEAD ABOVE WATER

In a society which wrenches mothers away from everything they are used to and shuts them into little boxes alone with their babies it isn't surprising that some women become depressed. Vivienne Welburn, in her book *Post Natal Depression* (see page 201), describes the dilemma vividly:

> *'After we have given birth it is as if we wake up to find that a mountain of sand has been deposited in front of the doors of our home. Some women get to work energetically to dig routes out. They have friends who come along to help. They work round the sand, and over the sand; they find marvellously inventive ways to cope with the situation. Some women stick to one route. Some try to dig their way out and get buried, others just look at it, feel defeated, retreat within their four walls and give up.'*

Talk to people with babies. They are probably feeling isolated too and just waiting for someone else to talk to them. In any new field of work it helps to find like-minded people to discuss your experience with. If you are a father taking the main responsibility for child care you may feel at a disadvantage in this female world. Changing social patterns (and unemployment) mean that many more men are child caring. Search them out. They will probably be as keen for company as you are.

Organise yourself with a bag containing everything your baby needs for trips. Keep it permanently supplied near the front door. Then add a fresh bottle if you need one and walk out with your baby when you want to.

Groups and meeting places to go to together (addresses on page 203)

Your local clinic or health centre may organise postnatal support or discussion groups.

Meet a Mum is a nationwide organisation started through an article in *Woman's Own*. It is particularly welcoming to new mothers who feel isolated and depressed, but any new mother can come and energetic members are always welcome for starting new groups.

The National Childbirth Trust organises postnatal support groups mainly for women who have already been to birth preparation classes in the area. You can contact the head office for your local organiser.

Social services should be able to provide a list of *One o'clock clubs* (these are informal groups where you can meet and chat with other new parents over a cup of tea).

Mother and toddler groups are open to people with babies too and they often organise activities such as health courses, sewing groups, toy making, child development and so on.

Family centres are open at any time for tea and company.

The local education authority should keep a list of courses which provide child care facilities. Here you can learn a new skill, broaden your mind, and meet new people, while your baby is looked after by an experienced crèche worker.

Community centres usually organise a variety of activities some of which are tailored to the needs of new mothers.

Starting your own group is not as hard as it sounds. Ask your GP or health visitor if you could put up a note on the wall during baby clinics. If they like the idea they may provide you with a place to meet at the health centre, perhaps during clinic time, or you could organise the first meeting at your own home.

Time for you

'He seemed to want constant attention, day and night. When he dropped off I would put him down and then just slump across the table thinking "please don't wake up". I would hear him cry and my whole body would scream "please please don't wake up." '

Many mothers drag themselves in a state of exhaustion from feed to change and expect (and are too often expected) to run the home, do the shopping, cook the evening meal and then have everything organised and tidy when their partner returns from work in the evening. Then it is far more likely to be him who nips down the pub for a pint, than her.

Among couples where the father takes the major share of child care, this pattern is less likely to be set. Barbara finds:

'When I get home at about 5.30, he is practically waiting in the hall with his coat on. He is off out for a quiet drink and a break after the pressures of the day. I don't mind, I know how much more tiring it is to care for a baby than to do a day's work at the office. Anyway, I enjoy the privacy, being alone with her after so many hours apart.'

Share the load If your baby is demanding and wakeful, by early evening you will be ready to drop. Since it is extremely unlikely that your partner's work is more gruelling than yours, try to set a pattern right from the start, in which the absent partner takes over child care at this time. It will give you time to relax, and your partner time to get to know the baby.

Baby swapping can give you a welcome break. It is particularly valuable for single parents. A friend with a baby of similar age can take yours on one day and then you take hers on

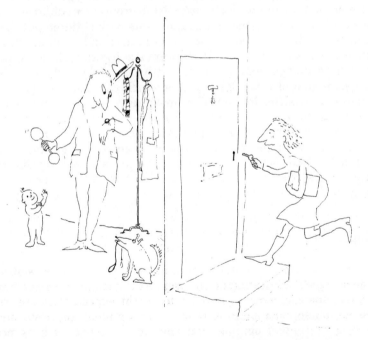

'When I get home at 5.30 he's practically waiting in the hall with his coat on. . . . He's off out for a quiet drink and a break. . . . I don't mind, I know how much more tiring it is to care for a baby than to do a day's work at the office.'

another. Start with just an hour or two to avoid feeding problems and then gradually increase the time. It really helps to make a regular arrangement rather than to leave it on a casual basis so that you can plan to make the most of your free time.

Of course you can include more than one baby. Maggie and her three friends organised a group every Thursday afternoon:

'At first there would always be two parents with the four babies but, as they got older, one parent could manage alone. The children became great friends and they still meet on Thursdays though they are now at school. They are happy with any of us and in any of our homes. They will even sleep overnight with each other which cuts down the babysitting problems. It is they who have benefited most. Especially the three who are only children.'

Babysitting circles may already exist in your area. Ask around neighbours with children, NCT groups, toy libraries and so on. You can start one yourself. Parents with children put their names on a list. One person acts as organiser and everyone starts off with a few points. Then, if you want a babysitter, the organiser finds a willing parent and you pay with points. If you then babysit for some one else you earn points which can then be spent on another babysitter for you. The job of organiser can be rotated to share the work.

Babysitters are usually passed on by word of mouth. A neighbour with teenage children is a good bet. Failing that, contact a local school and ask if there are any willing and responsible sixth-formers. Make sure that your sitters know what to do if the baby wakes, and how to find you in an emergency.

Separation

There have always been different and conflicting theories about the best way of bringing up children. At the moment women tend to find themselves in a real bind. On the one hand, more and more women are returning to work, on the other, there is still a strong current of opinion that says mothers should keep pre-school children with them all the time.

Since the 1950s mothers have been plagued with guilt about the damage which they can do to their children by leaving them for periods of time. The so-called evidence has been taken from

the troubled lives of babies separated from their parents because
of government evacuation policies in wartime. The difficulty that
these babies and young children felt in adjusting to life with
strange people in strange places cannot in any way be compared
to separation on a daily basis. Even the smallest babies will
settle down quite happily with an alternative carer if they are
introduced to the idea gradually, and at the right time.

If you wait until your baby is nearing eight months you will
have a problem on your hands. At about that stage your baby
will suddenly realise that you are not attached to her by a piece
of string, she can lose you. If you start leaving her with someone
else now she will be frightened and find it very hard to settle. It
is best, particularly if you want to leave her regularly, to get her
used to the person who will be looking after her well before the
eight-month stage and preferably before six months so that her
alternative carers will be part of the secure world which she
already knows.

Of course all children have different personalities. Some will
always find it hard to settle in unfamiliar surroundings, whereas
others seem impervious to changes in routine. Here are some
suggestions from parents who have gone through it.

* Let her get to know her new carer in your company first.
* Leave her for a few short breaks to start with.
* If she cries at first, don't be deterred. Some babies take
  longer to settle than others. You may find that she stops
  crying the minute you leave and doesn't start again until
  you return. Just persevere, as regularly as you can manage,
  until she gets used to it.
* If she cries all the time when you leave her for one hour, try
  leaving her for two hours. This may seem cruel but it is just
  possible that you are being over-anxious and not giving her
  a chance to settle and get to know her new carer.
* Let her know when you are leaving and then leave quickly
  and cheerfully. Some people feel that it is easier just to slip
  out quietly. Your child may seem less concerned at first, but
  only because she hasn't noticed your absence. Once she re-
  alises you have disappeared she may feel even more worried.
  Be brave, say goodbye, grit your teeth against the cries, and
  then leave quickly. Don't change your mind and stop to
  comfort her. It will only draw out the agony. Nine times out

of ten she will have turned her mind to other things within minutes of your departure.
* If you are returning to work and it is very important that your baby settles, you will feel anxious. That anxiety will be transmitted to your baby and you may well find that, on your last joint visits to the minder, she will cry and be unsettled. Once you have left, she will probably relax and start to take in her new environment.

Love hurts you too

Separation anxiety does not only affect babies. Mothers feel it too.

'I knew I needed a break. I was ground down and exhausted and I just could not work out why my baby seemed so difficult to please. Friends would drop by and offer to take him for a few hours and I would always invent an excuse. I could not bear to part with him. It was like having a painful leg. I didn't like the pain but my leg is part of me. I didn't want it chopped off either. After a few months I found that I could leave him with my mum for an hour or two without eating my heart out. Then gradually I relaxed and found that I could let go without coming to any harm. Looking back, after a year, I can hardly believe that I could have let myself drown like that.'

This fiercely protective feeling towards your baby is as important to her survival as the antibodies in your breast milk. A tiny, vulnerable creature who can do nothing for herself needs protection. We can only presume that this feeling of protection for small creatures is built deep into our psyches. Advertising exploits that 'aaahh' feeling that most of us have towards babies for all its worth. Pictures of kittens, puppies, little chicks, and babies are regularly churned out by tabloid newspapers in order to increase sales.

When the baby is your own, and you are directly responsible for her survival, that feeling grows and you may feel as though it is taking you over. When you feel like this you are also very vulnerable.

'I had always known that I would want, and need, to go back to work. An old friend came to visit and started parroting nonsense about babies needing their mothers and sometimes not being ready to leave even by school age. I was torn with

guilt. Her words haunted me. Now, three years later, I can tell
her that she was wrong but when you have only just had your
baby you believe anything.'

If you have made an agreement to share her care, or you intend
to return to work, you may find the first parting pretty painful.
Elana returned to work when her two sons were 6 and four and
a half months old:

'When they first went to the minder I felt destroyed for about a
week. They were fine, but I found it very difficult to let go.
Still, I knew that for two days a week and the beginning and
end of each day I could be a good mother. For seven days I
can't.'

Carol's baby was five months old:

'The initial separation was traumatic for me. Throughout that
long morning, I was pining and dabbing away at my eyes,
resisting the temptation to ring the nursery. I had tried
unsuccessfully to wean him on to a bottle so at lunchtime I
ran all the way there to feed him. When I arrived he had
already had a bottle and was perfectly happy.'

There is no way of avoiding these pangs. Just as you feel bad if
your lover departs for a long period of time you will feel the
wrench when the extraordinary intimacy of those first months is
broken for the first time. You can only try and ensure that your
baby is being well cared for.

If you go through a bad patch when your baby doesn't want
to settle you will feel guilty. It is at a time like this that punitive
attitudes really bite. Remember that there is a baby care expert
to support every possible variety of child care theory. Here is a
pleasantly reassuring thought from 'expert' Ronald Schaffer's
book *Mothering*:

'There is no need to prolong the controversy about whether the
mother must be the infant's constant companion throughout
each twenty-four hour day. Clearly some minimum period of
togetherness is required but . . . it is the personal qualities
that the adult brings to the interaction that matters most. . . .
There is no reason why mother and child should not spend a
portion of the day apart.'

The first day back at work

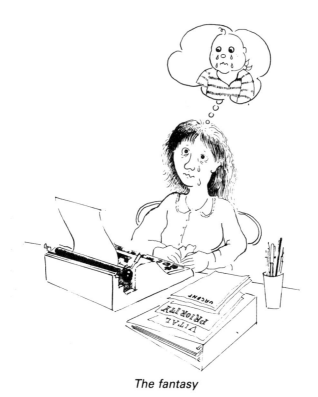

The fantasy

Back to work

If you are already back in paid work or looking for a job by the time your baby is eight months old you are in good company. In ten years, between 1971 and 1981, the number of women back in work or looking for jobs, at least part-time, rose from 9 per cent to 25 per cent.

The speed of this increase has meant that women have had very little time in which to pass on information about the best ways of finding child care and balancing the demands of bringing up children with a job.

You cannot expect much help from the state. The official line from successive governments has been that women with children

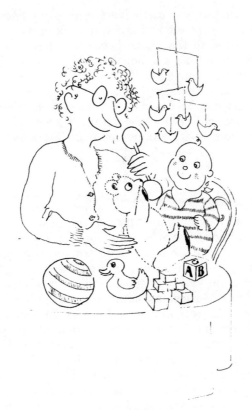

The reality

under school age should stay at home with them. It has been easier to label women who disobey as irresponsible than to spend money in providing the high quality child care that so many more children now need.

The result is that parents are very much on their own when looking for someone to care for their children. The majority depend on friends, relations, or work back-to-back shifts with their partners. For those women whose wages will stretch, these are the alternatives:

Mother substitutes

Childminders are registered and can be contacted through your local social services department. If you can afford, or have space for, *live in help* you can advertise through *The Lady* (see page 204). An *au pair* would do, if you work part-time (au pair agencies are listed in the phone book) but they should not be expected to do more than five hours' work each day. If you want someone to come to your home daily you could advertise locally. Registration is not necessary. *Nanny sharing* may be a good option. A nanny can be based at one house, and then care for two, or even three children whose parents then divide her wages and expenses. Some NCT groups (see page 204) organise nanny sharing lists.

Groups

Nursery care is not widely available for babies, but check with social services for local day nurseries. If you are single you would get priority in a *council day nursery*. In some urban areas *community nurseries* have been set up. They may have long waiting lists but provide model care (small-scale, parent- and staff-controlled, non-sexist and non-racist, combining education with care and usually heavily subsidised), so it is worth the wait. *Workplace nurseries* are occasionally provided in large establishments and some *private nurseries* do cater for babies but they may be expensive and are often understaffed (ideally you should have a ratio of three under-two's to one staff member).

If you would like your baby to have the benefit of group care but cannot get a nursery place, you could set up a *child care group*. This works best for part-time workers who can join a child care rota. Like nanny sharing, five or six parents then employ one nursery worker between them, providing space in one house (or rotating the house monthly) and sharing costs. If you live on an estate, you could ask for the use of an unoccupied flat for a child care group.

Keeping life in perspective

The first few months of your first baby's life are a series of crises. No sooner have you stopped worrying whether or not she will keep breathing through the night then you are agonising over when she will stop waking you. If you get over that hurdle (some of us are still waiting) you find yourself sick with anxiety over the texture of the mashed bananas you should be feeding her. It is perhaps reassuring to keep in mind that most children are out of nappies, eating solids, talking and walking by the time they reach school, no matter how their parents mashed the bananas.

USEFUL BOOKS AND PAMPHLETS

All About Twins: A Handbook for Parents, Gillian Leigh, Routledge & Kegan Paul, 1983 (£4.95.)

Bargaining Report 8, Labour Research Department, 78 Blackfriars Road, London SE1.

Employment Rights for the Expectant Mother, from Department of Employment Offices (free).

The Experience of Breastfeeding, Sheila Kitzinger, Penguin, 1979 (£1.79).

The Experience of Infertility, Naomi Pfeffer and Anne Woollett, Virago, 1983 (£3.50).

From Here to Maternity, Anne Oakley, Penguin, 1979 (£2.25), interviews.

Guide to Maternity Rights, available from all Department of Health and Social Security Offices (free).

The Herpes Manual, Carol Woddis and Sue Blanks, Wigmore, 1983 (£2.99).

The Home Birth Handbook, Monaco and Junor, 1980, from The Manor House, Thelnetham, near Diss, Norfolk (£2.80 including postage).

Let's Have Healthy Children, Adele Davis, Allen & Unwin, 1981 (£1.95), nutritional advice for pregnant women.

Maternity Rights for Working Women, Jean Coussins, National Council for Civil Liberties, 21 Tabard Street, London SE1 (75p).

The New Good Birth Guide, Sheila Kitzinger, Penguin, 1983 (£3.95), a guide to the best hospitals for having your baby.

Nurseries Now, Hughes and Mayall, Penguin, 1980 (£1.95), a helpful and reassuring book for mothers who intend to return to work.

The Place of Birth, ed. Sheila Kitzinger and John Davis, Oxford University Press (£15.00 hardback, £10.50 paper).

Post Natal Depression, Vivienne Welburn, Fontana, 1980 (£1.25).

Self Insemination, from Sisterwrite, 190 Upper Street, London N1 (£1.50).

When Pregnancy Fails, Judith Borg and Susan Lasker, Routledge & Kegan Paul, 1982 (£3.95), a supportive book for parents who have suffered miscarriage or still birth.

Your Social Security, Frances Bennett, Penguin, 1982 (£1.95), a guide to benefits.

USEFUL ORGANISATIONS

Association for Improvements in Maternity Services (AIMS) is a campaigning organisation with a bimonthly newsletter. Write to Elizabeth Key, Goose Green Barn, Much Hoole, Preston, Lancashire PR4 4TD.

Association for Post Natal Illness, 7 Gowan Avenue, London SE6 provides telephone counselling for mothers with postnatal depression. Write and you will be contacted immediately.

Association of Radical Midwives (ARMS), 88 The Drive, London SW20, is for midwives – they may be able to put you in touch with an independent midwife in your area.

Association for Smoking and Health (ASH), 27 Mortimer Street, London W11, will give you help in stopping smoking.

British Acupuncture Association, 34 Alderney Street, London SW1, lists qualified practitioners and provides information about acupuncture. Send £1.50 and SAE.

British Homeopathic Association, 27a Devonshire Street, London W1N 1RJ, provides lists of registered medical practitioners.

British Hypnotherapy Association, 67 Upper Berkeley Street, London W1H 7DH, lists registered practitioners with information about their qualifications. Send £1 and SAE.

British Pregnancy Advisory Service, Guildhall Buildings, Navigation Street, Birmingham B2 4BT (021–643 1461), will tell you where your nearest advice centre is.

Centre for Advice on Natural Alternatives (CANA), Tyddyn y Mynydd, Llanelly Hill, Gwent.

The Compassionate Friends, c/o 5 Lower Clifton Hill, Bristol 8 (0272–292 778), is a self-help network of parents who help each other through the crisis of still birth or infant death.

DAWN, c/o Ruth Joicey, St Clement's DDA, 2a Bow Road, London E3, is an organisation to help women who drink.

Hyperactive Children's Support Group, c/o Mrs Colquhoun, Mayfield House, Yapton Road, Barnham, Bognor Regis, West Sussex.

The Job Sharing Project, 347a Upper Street, London N1 0PD, will give advice to job sharers.

The Lady, 40 Bedford Street, London WC2, is a magazine which lists adverts for, and from, nannies.

Maternity Alliance, 309 Kentish Town Road, London NW5 2TJ, campaigns for improved maternity rights and provides information on rights at work.

Meet a Mum, c/o Mary Whitlock, 26a Cumnor Hill, Oxford, organises groups nationwide for new mums who feel isolated and want a bit of company and support.

National Childbirth Trust, 9 Queensborough Terrace, London W2 (01–221 3833), has a nationwide network of childbirth preparation teachers, postnatal support groups and breastfeeding counsellors.

National Childcare Campaign, c/o Surrey Docks Childcare Project, Docklands Settlement, Redriff Road, London SE16, campaigns for better nursery facilities.

National Childminders' Association, 13 London Road, Bromley, Kent BR1 1DE, supports childminders and can give you information about their rights and responsibilities, and yours.

Pre-Eclamptic Toxaemia Society (PETS), c/o Dawn James, 88 Plumberrow, Lee Chapel North, Basildon, Essex SS15 5LP, is a self-help society for women suffering high blood pressure in pregnancy.

The Sickle Cell Society, c/o Brent Community Health Council, 16 High Street, London NW10, and *The Sickle Cell Centre* (01–459 1292, ext. 235), provide advice and counselling for women with this disease.

Society to Support Home Confinements, c/o Margaret Whyte, 17 Laburnum Avenue, Durham City, Co. Durham.

Still Birth and Perinatal Death Association, c/o 66 Harley Street, London W1N 1AE, gives support to parents.

INDEX

passim means here and there throughout